I love how Nikki talks about aging and how it is more than saggy skin, wrinkles and gray hair. She actually explains what is happening to us on the inside during the aging process, not just what is happening on the outside. Very useful information provided to help slow down the aging process from the inside. Great book!

Ann McIndoo

Incredible book with new and fresh information on controlling the aging process. I especially like how the author says to imagine ourselves in our 90's being mentally sharp, spirited and strong with no aches and pains or prescription medicines. She has definitely planted a seed in my mind that this is how life could be at 90. My previous mindset was that I would end up with lots of aches and pains and probably with Alzheimer's! Found all the anti-aging strategies in Nikki's book very helpful.

Katie Rodgers

There is an entire chapter devoted to the power of food and how it affects our behavior, moods and aging. The idea of "healing foods" is presented and many examples given. There is also a section on how to detox your body from the old way of eating. After reading this book I have decided to change the way I eat and follow some of the guidelines in Nikki's book.

Phil Solis

I spent lots of time and money attending various workshops and classes over the years and Nikki has successfully condensed all that valuable information into her easy to read book.

E.J. Wright

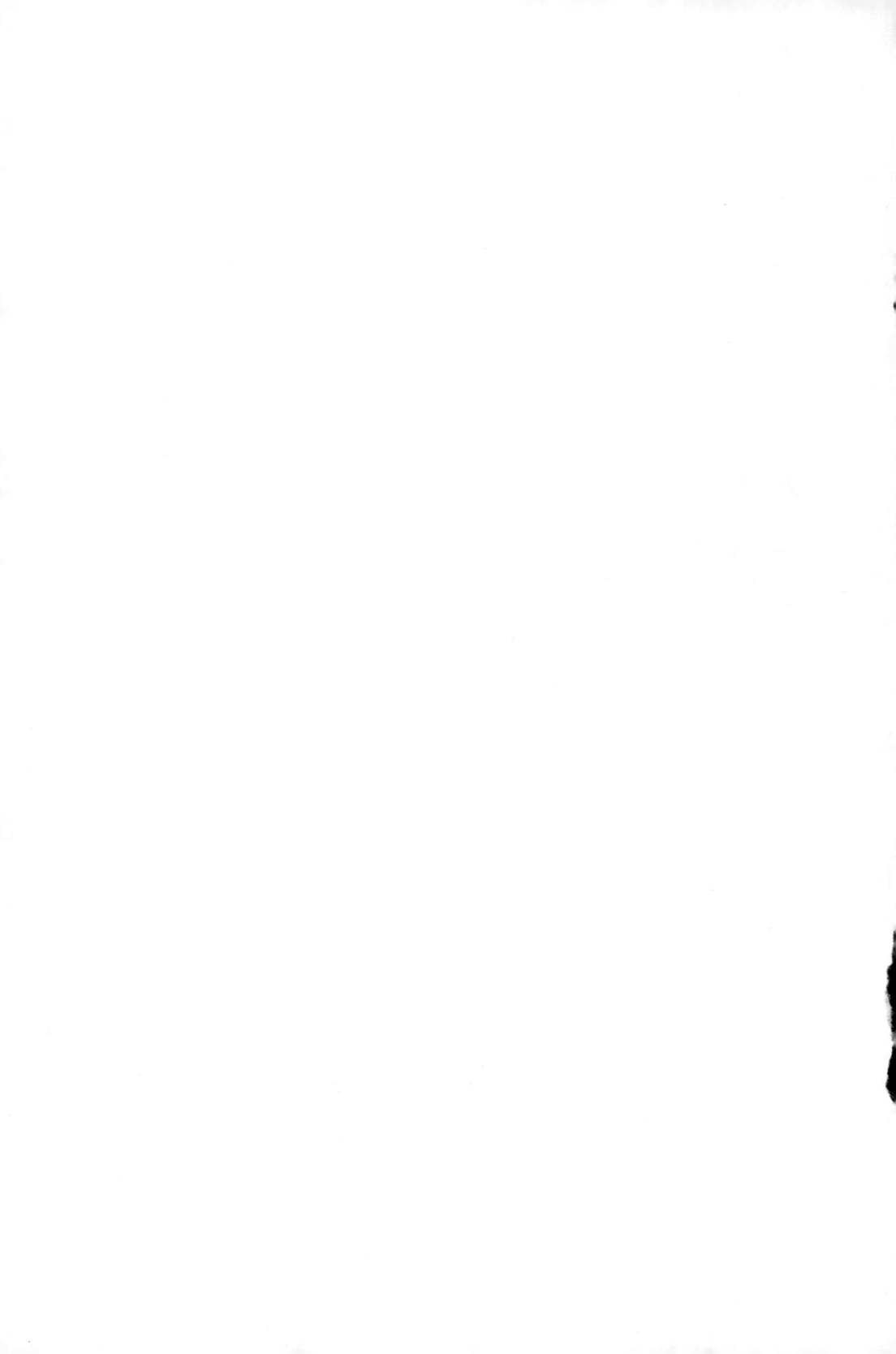

The Anti-Aging Body

60 Days To A Sexier, Younger, Healthier New You!

NIKKI STEWART

ISBN: 978-1-941142-54-7

Medical Disclaimer
This book has been written and published strictly for informational and educational purposes only. It is not intended to serve as medical advice or to be any form of medical treatment. You should always consult with your physician before altering or changing any aspect of your medical treatment. Do not stop or change any prescription medications without the guidance and advice of your physician. Any use of the information in this book is made on the reader's good judgment and is the reader's sole responsibility. This book is not intended to diagnose or treat any medical condition and is not a substitute for a physician.

DEDICATION

"Love wholeheartedly, be surprised, give thanks and praise—then you will discover the fullness of your life."
—Brother David Steindl-Rast

This book is dedicated to the two most amazing souls on this earth, Melody Joy and Matthew Jonathan. I treasure and love you both with my whole heart and soul. You are my inspiration and motivation for all I have accomplished in this life. You have made my life worth living, adding rich color and texture to the fabric of my life. You have made me a better person. I am honored to be your mother and am so proud of both of you.

ACKNOWLEDGEMENTS

I could not have written this book without the help of my assistant, Melody Morales. I am truly grateful for your daily support, keeping me on task and making everything run smoothly.

Special gratitude to all my friends and family who have touched my life in unique and special ways. Elizabeth Wright, Phil Solis and Catherine Veritas, thank you for believing in me and encouraging me to follow my dreams. You have made me who I am today.

And, of course, Ann McIndoo, my Author's Coach, who got this book out of my head and into my hands.

Contents

INTRODUCTION

M ost people I meet are on a quest for the ever-elusive fountain of youth. They look in the mirror. and hardly recognize the person staring back at them. Who is that person with the sagging skin? Who is that person with the gray hair? Those wrinkles weren't there yesterday!

I also know people who consistently lie about their age. With technology advancing as fast as it is, there are so many "solutions" to the aging process. There is plastic surgery, hair dye, botox, and an endless array of fillers. There seems to be new products coming out on a daily basis that promise younger looking skin or a more youthful appearance. Foundation with nanoparticles will hide your "flaws." Or, a silicone face cream promises to fill in uneven texture. Because we want so desperately to believe these claims, we buy the latest and greatest product or device. Unfortunately, we end up with an empty wallet and a drawer full of empty promises.

There are also those people I meet who have given up. I am saddened when I meet someone who thinks that feeling good about they way they look is not in the cards for them. They don't take pride in their appearance, nor in how they feel.

The bottom line is that we all want to feel good about ourselves. We want to be happy with our appearance. Let's face it, when we feel good about our appearance, the rest of our life seems a bit brighter. I find that, whoever I am talking to, they want to feel good, inside and out. It is universal.

One thing I have noticed is that most people want an easy fix. They want that magic pill that will do the trick. Truth be told, I would like that magic pill, too. But, it simply does not exist. There are simple answers, but no easy answers. To achieve the anti-aging body, we must change our lifestyle.

I take a global approach to developing the anti-aging body. The fountain of youth is not found in a pill, procedure or even a diet plan. It is found in developing a lifestyle, a mindset that puts you on the right track. It is most certainly is found in what you feed your body and your mind. But, it is also found in how you take care of your body on a daily basis, by honoring your need for rest, for exercise and play.

I have discovered in my own life that looking good and feeling good starts from within. I ask myself some simple questions throughout the day: What is my mindset? How do I want to feel? How you feel, both emotionally and physically, does show up on the outside. Am I living congruent with my goals? Are the daily choices I make moving me toward my ultimate goal? These are questions I have learned to ask myself in every area of my life.

In regard to developing the anti-aging body, these questions are crucial. Is indulging in that bag of chips going to make me feel good? Am I eating them because I am feeling down or depressed? We all know that it won't make me look good! I have also learned that we do not live in a vacuum. What is good for me in one area of my life, is good for me across the board. If I have a sweet tooth and I indulge in candy, it won't nourish me physically and chances are I will be eating a shit storm of chemicals and preservatives. After I indulged, I may feel guilty or defeated.

However, if I eat a piece of raw chocolate or a bowl of fresh berries, I will have consumed a good portion of anti-oxidants and micronutrients and will nourish my body. I know that I am moving in the right direction towards my goal - a healthy, vibrant body.

I have also discovered that everything is made up of vibrational energy. If one wants to look good and feel good, one must make a concerted effort to raise their vibrational energy. In fact, science has proven what the wisdom of the ages has taught for millennia. Everything has vibrational energy. When you feel good about yourself, you feel happier and you raise your vibrational energy. You are likely to make choices that will benefit you in all areas of your life, including food and exercise choices. The opposite is also true. If you don't feel good about yourself, you lower your vibrational energy. You are then likely to make choices that you will later regret.

Albert Einstein said that "Everything is energy and that is all there is to it. Match the frequency of the reality you want and you cannot help but to get that reality. It can be no other way. This is not philosophy, this is physics."

You may be thinking two questions at this point. How do I raise my vibrational energy? And, what does this have to do with aging anyway? Bear with me as I explain.

Look at what you put in your mouth. What is its vibrational energy? Is it alive and vibrant? Or, is it a food-like product with no vitality to it? Look at your body care products. What are their vibrational energy? Are they made up of chemicals you cannot pronounce? Or, are they made from natural, health-producing ingredients? As we will discuss later in the book, the vibrational energy of things and emotions can be measured. Are you bringing down your vibrational energy without even knowing it?

Are you working hard at trying to change your lifestyle, but not able to sustain it? This book seeks to partner with you as you develop a lifestyle that truly serves you and helps you to achieve the anti-aging body you deserve. Whatever your desire in picking up this book, applying the principles within will enhance the quality of your life.

CHAPTER ONE

The Anti-Aging Body

─────────────────────────────────

"Your body is a temple, but only if you treat it as one."
~Astrid Alauda

D o you feel like you are getting old? Do you look in the mirror and notice a wrinkle or two that you would swear weren't there yesterday? Do you look in the mirror and wonder who is the person staring back at you? You feel young inside, but the mirror tells a different story. What is aging anyway?

To understand the concept of anti-aging, it is important to understand a bit about the aging process. Once we understand how and why we age, we can then figure out what to do about it.

The question is, what is aging? It is more than getting wrinkles, sagging skin and gray hair. These are the readily apparent manifestations of aging and the great news is we can cover these up - we can dye our hair and have plastic surgery. Unfortunately, this does absolutely nothing to slow the aging process. Aging is much more than what happens to us on the outside.

The following definition from the Concise Encyclopedia states aging is the:

"Gradual change in an organism that leads to increased risk of weakness, disease, and death. It takes place in a cell, an organ, or the total organism over the entire adult life span of any living thing. There is a decline in biological functions and in ability to adapt to metabolic stress. Overall effects of aging include reduced immunity, loss of muscle strength, decline in memory and other aspects of cognition, and loss of colour in the hair and elasticity in the skin. In women, the process accelerates after menopause."

This definition begs the question of how that gradual change in an organism starts? In this book, I will get to the root cause of aging and provide you with a system to stack the deck in your favor in fighting the *aging process.*

I invite you to close your eyes and picture a 90 year old in your mind. Describe their appearance. Are they frail, barely holding on in a convalescent hospital? Are they stricken with diseases such as Alzheimer's disease or dementia and taking numerous prescription medication? Or, are they healthy, vibrant and an active member of society?

Almost guaranteed, the image you held in your mind is exactly where you are headed. Is that a scary thought for you? If you do not believe that 90 year-olds can be healthy and vital, enjoying their lives to the fullest, you will not be headed in that direction. Let's change that! Let's design a system that will allow you to enjoy your life to the fullest, all the days of your life.

I talk to too many people who think that aches and pains, dementia and disease are just a normal, natural part of getting old. These are not normal, inevitable, albeit unpleasant, conditions associated with aging. Health is your birthright, no matter your age. You can be healthy and vital well into your 90s. I want you to form a picture in your mind of a mentally sharp, spirited, strong 90-year-old version of you. No aches, no pains, no prescription medication. And, no disease. Hold that image in your mind when you wake up in the morning and before falling asleep at night. That image will direct where you will be going.

"The doctor of the future will no longer treat the human frame with drugs, but rather will cure and prevent disease with nutrition."

~Thomas Edison

Your body is a masterpiece. It is a finely tuned machine. It is exquisite. It is performing exactly as it should. But, you may thinking, what about me? I have diabetes? Or heart disease? Or osteoporosis? Or auto-immune disorders? Or arthritis? Are you saying my body is functioning properly?

My answer is "YES!" Based upon the fuel you give your body, the thoughts you think, your level of exercise, the amount of sleep and recovery you give your body, it is functioning exactly as designed.

Your body is in a constant state of flux, attempting to achieve homeostasis. Its number one function is to keep you alive.

Let's take the example of osteoporosis. Your blood's pH level must stay within a very narrow range, from 7.35 to 7.45, or you will die. If your body is overly acidic due to your lifestyle, it will leach calcium out of your bones to bring the blood's pH into proper balance. Over time, your bones will become weak and osteoporosis will develop.

Osteoporosis, in this example, is not a function of aging even though many people of advanced years have this condition. Nor is it a matter of your body not functioning properly. It is a function of your body functioning exactly as it should, given what you have fed it. It is your body's attempt to keep itself alive and protect itself from overly acidic blood pH. The question to ask is, how did your body develop this acidic state in the first place? Are you eating foods that become acidic in your body? Are you eating processed foods? Are you in a constant state of stress? Are you too busy to exercise?

Let's get back to the questions of what causes aging and what can you do about it. Chronic inflammation and oxidation (or free radical damage) are at the root of aging. Inflammation and oxidation are caused by stress. Stress is stress, whether it is caused by the foods you eat, the thoughts you think or due to an injury you suffered. When inflammation or oxidation become chronic, it impairs our ability to deal with stress. The stress becomes chronic, leading to more inflammation and oxidation. It is a vicious cycle. The good news is that it is a vicious cycle that can be broken!

It is imperative to learn to work with the body. The human body has the innate wisdom to heal, when given proper nutrients and the ability to properly eliminate. Again, keep in mind, your body is functioning exactly as it is designed, given the fuel you give it. What can be done on a daily basis to reverse the aging process? The answer is: EATING!

That's right. Something as simple and ordinary as eating directly impacts every aspect of the aging process. Those hamburgers and French fries cause oxidation and inflammation and accelerate the aging process.

To begin developing your personalized Anti-Aging Body, here are ten simple and basic guidelines:

#1 - If you don't know what is in your food, don't buy it. If man made it, it probably won't benefit your health. If you can't pronounce the word on the food label, put it back on the shelf. Eliminate food dyes, preservatives or artificial sweeteners.

#2 - Eat organic. Conventionally grown foods are grown with petroleum based pesticides and herbicides. Pesticides function in different ways, but one of the most common and effective methods is to cause nerve damage to the insect. Fruits and vegetables are doused with such chemicals. The food, soil and water become contaminated. These chemicals can build up in your fatty tissues, including your brain! So, opt for organic!

#3 - Eliminate gluten from your diet. The bread of today is a far cry from the bread of just 40 years ago. Gluten can affect your thyroid for up to 6 months after eating that cookie. Many people experience Celiac's Disease, while others suffer from Non-Gluten Celiac Sensitivity (NGCS). NGCS can lead to a whole host of autoimmune conditions.

#4 - Your body will thank you if you swear off all added sugars and artificial sweeteners. Start with high fructose corn syrup! HFCS is wrong in so many ways. It is derived from corn, and the corn used is almost guaranteed to be genetically modified (GMO). HFCS is a highly processed industrial "food" that is foreign to the body, thus it is toxic. Your body does not know how to process it. It triggers insulin spikes and results in the development of metabolic disorders and obesity. Don't stop at HFCS! Eliminate all added sweeteners. Ditching the soda is a great first step. Soda is contaminated with either artificial sweeteners or high fructose corn syrup (HFCS). Artificial sweeteners such as aspartame are neurotoxins. In other words, it is toxic to your body and your brain!

#5 - Never eat anything that has been genetically modified (GMO). At this time there are no laws requiring foods to be labeled if they contain GMOs. Read the labels. High risk crops include alfalfa, canola, corn, cotton papaya, soy, sugar beets, zucchini and yellow summer squash. If the product contains anything made from these high risk crops, put it back on the shelf. It is safest to opt for 100% organic.

#6 - Drink plenty of fresh, spring water. Water is the great lubricant. Your body is, or should be, about 70% water. You cannot survive long without water. It also dissolves and flushes out toxins. Since we are bombarded with toxins from our environment and our food, it is imperative we flush them out with fresh spring water. A rule of thumb is to drink 1/2 your weight in ounces each day.

#7 - Supplement with enzymes. Enzymes are the spark of life. Without enzymes you die. There are metabolic enzymes and digestive enzymes. Taking digestive enzymes with each meal ensures that your body is able to break down the food you consume: proteins to amino acids; fats to fatty acids; and carbohydrates to glucose. All elements your body needs to perform at its best. I provide my clients with professional grade enzymes, you can also find them at www.Anti-AgingBody.com.

#8 - Incorporate plenty of fresh, green leafy veggies in your diet. A great way to get several servings a day is to make yourself a delicious green smoothie every day.

#9 - Eat an antioxidant rich diet. We lead such stress-filled lives. Stress leads to inflammation. To counter the effects of inflammation, it is important to eat a diet rich in antioxidants. Look for colorful fruits and vegetables. Berries, red and orange bell pepper, cherries and raw cacao are some of my favorites.

#10 - Develop a healthy lifestyle. Take the time to nurture your body by getting adequate sleep, exercise and sunshine. Love deeply, laugh often and enjoy nature. Make the effort to develop healthy relationships.

I am personally committed to helping you shatter that old stereotype of a broken-down 90 year old. I am dedicated to helping you reclaim your youth and feel great to the very end of your life. It is fun to develop your own Anti-Aging Body, a system or game plan that works for you, based upon the principles in this book.

Yes, in as short as 60 days, you can have a sexier, younger, healthier new You - no matter your age.

CHAPTER TWO

My Story

"Food is powerful medicine. You can eat yourself to health."
Nikki Jeannine Stewart

I grew up in a suburb of Los Angeles in the 1980's. My mother was a registered nurse and my father was an attorney. After my parents got married and my mother had my oldest brother, she decided to stay at home to raise six kids; I was number five of six. Ultimately, I followed my father's footsteps and became an attorney too.

Being the daughter of a registered nurse, I was taught to trust the medical profession, believing doctors had the wisdom and the knowledge to heal the body. It seemed that even though there was a huge emphasis on education in our family, I checked my common sense at the door and blindly trusted my doctor with my health and my life.

When I was 11 years old I suffered from severe intestinal pain. My mother took me to the doctor. We described my symptoms and I walked away with a prescription. He put me on a phenobarbital prescription medication along with an over-the-counter medication. As an adult, I was curious about that prescription. I discovered that the side effects of phenobarbital can include severe seizures and even death. I was stunned that a doctor would even think of putting a child on such a strong medication, especially when my mother and I had only spent a few minutes with him describing my symptoms.

No one took the time to discuss my diet. No one asked me what was going on in my life. The pill was the answer. Yes, it did help alleviate the pain, temporarily. But the symptoms continued off and on throughout the years. It definitely did not cure me.

Years later I suffered from a "flu" that just wouldn't get better. My doctor could not figure out what was wrong with me even after a battery of tests. At first he suspected Lupus. I was only 21 years old at the time and I had never even heard of that word before! I was scared and knew no other way than to trust my doctor. He held the key to healing my body - or so I thought.

When it turned out I did not have Lupus, he then thought maybe I was suffering from tuberculosis of my intestine. I did not even know you could get tuberculosis in your intestines. When that test was negative, he suspected cancer! So imagine, I am 21 years old, I have my whole life ahead of me and I am being faced with the prospect of having one of many debilitating and possibly fatal diseases.

My boyfriend and my grandmother were with me through this process but I still felt really alone and scared. I was being led down a bewildering and unknown path which was full of invasive tests and procedure after procedure. I did not know any other way. I trusted my doctor would get to the root of the problem. It was what I had been raised to believe. I just went to the doctor when I had something wrong with me and he figured out the problem. He would write a prescription and the symptoms would go away.

That wasn't happening this time. Even though I was taught to simply trust the guy in the white coat it was becoming clear that he did not know what was going on. Doubts were starting to creep in. He put me on powerful steroids to cut down the inflammation. He never explained to me what steroids were nor how to take them. I was just told to take them. And, just like a good little girl, I took them.

About the time I was about to receive the diagnosis of Crohn's disease, I went to my chiropractor. In passing I had mentioned to him what I had been going through. He almost yelled at me for not coming to him first. He actually took the time to talk to me! He explained to me how the body worked and that one organ system does not live in a vacuum unaffected by other organ systems. He explained the dangers and side effects of the steroids. He explained how the body has the innate wisdom to heal, when you give the body what it needs. First, I needed to stop toxifying my body. Then, I needed to start detoxifying my body.

He suggested I start taking chlorophyll which is an extremely nutrient dense, high vibration food and digestive enzymes. Miraculously, in just a few months, my body healed, just like he said it would! I have never had a flare up since.

I was disillusioned by my medical doctor and how he so cavalierly experimented with my health and my life. I was not up for exposing myself to that again, at least not any time soon.

A few years later I became pregnant with my daughter. I knew that pregnancy was not a disease and a hospital was not the place for my child to be born. I was young and healthy. I searched for a midwife and was lucky to find two amazing women who had a midwifery practice near my home. They were warm, nurturing and caring.

At the same time, I had a back-up plan if complications arose and I needed medical intervention. I made sure my medical care provider had records on my pregnancy. I went to the obstetrician for my regular appointments. He could not believe that I would even consider having a home birth! He did his best to scare me into having a hospital birth, telling me horror story after horror story.

He did me the biggest favor when he encouraged me to go to the maternity ward and see how nice and beautiful it was. I got off the elevator and there was a woman who was giving birth. I had heard the nurses encouraging her to push. I heard her husband talking to her. I heard the sounds of the monitors. The thing that really freaked me out was that she had not made a noise, not even a peep! Although I had never had a baby before, I watched enough TV and movies to know that the mother is usually making some noise.

It scared me to death! I knew that poor woman was so drugged up that she could not feel a thing. Right then and there that affirmed me that I was doing the right thing. Pregnancy was not a disease. My home was the best and safest place for my baby to be born.

I knew I wanted my baby to have the best possible start in life as possible. I had the most beautiful birth experience with both my daughter and my son. I would not have changed a thing.

You would think that after my experience with doctors that I would have been completely resistant to trusting that guy in the white coat again.

Unfortunately I was not. When my kids were in high school I began suffering from extreme fatigue. I would hit a wall every day. I just could not make it through the day without taking a nap. Sometimes it was only 20 minutes; sometimes I napped up to two hours. And it was becoming debilitating.

It got so bad that I finally succumbed to going to the doctor. He took my medical history and said he was going to try a couple of things. He told me I was not depressed but he thought maybe antidepressants (SSRI) would help me by lifting the fatigue. I was desperate to have energy again. Surely, this man in the white coat would have the answer to my problem. So like a good girl I took them for about 30 days.

There was no change. I went back to the doctor for my follow-up appointment, he looked at my chart, he looked at me and said, "You are not depressed, why are you taking these?" I could not believe that this man was experimenting with these potent drugs. I could not believe that he did not remember his thought process and reasons for putting me on this powerful medication.

He was playing with my life giving me pills that carry a black box warning. The black box warning is the strongest warning that the FDA requires. It is reserved for drugs that carry a significant risk of serious or life-threatening adverse effects. In the case of antidepressants, there is a risk of suicide and death. Needless to say, I never returned to that doctor again.

Several years later my brother was diagnosed with Celiac's disease. I thought that this might be the root of my fatigue. I went to another doctor to get tested except this doctor refused to test me because he said the condition was so rare he did not want to waste the insurance company's money.

I insisted on a bone density scan because one of the consequences of Celiac's disease is osteoporosis and several members of my immediate family had osteoporosis. The scan indicated that I had osteopenia. I felt I was too young to be old! I refused to go on medication. Instead, I educated myself on how to treat this condition. I started exercising with weights, changed my lifestyle and diet

By changing my diet and incorporating an exercise regimen, my fatigue lifted and my osteopenia vanished!

I was reminded that our bodies possess the innate wisdom and ability to heal. I realized that when we are experiencing symptoms they should be embraced. Our symptoms are there to tell us that something needs attention. They are our body's way of talking to us.

I also learned that bodies are functioning exactly the way that they were designed. They are behaving exactly as they should given the fuel that you give it. If you are experiencing any unwanted symptoms take a step back and look at what you are feeding yourself. But, keep in mind, you are feeding yourself more than just the physical food you eat.

When I was about 20 I had a job that I loved. For the most part, I enjoyed the people and the work. I was in school and everything was looking great. I started getting an itchy, blotchy rash; it was annoying and nothing made it go away. In fact it was just getting worse. I took a week off for vacation and went to Hawaii with some friends.

At the end of the week I realized I was completely symptom free. I went back to work on the next Monday, I got on the elevator, pushed the button and as I rode up to the sixth floor the itching and the redness immediately came back, with a vengeance! I had my rash all over again. For the first time, I had made the connection between stress and symptoms I was experiencing. I had never realized how powerfully stress impacted my life.

You see, my boss had been making advances toward me for the month or two prior to my vacation. He was married with two small children but he made it clear that he wanted to pursue an affair. I was completely distraught and did not know what to do and I did not have the tools or life skills to deal with the situation.

This was long before there were any lawsuits or any talk about sexual harassment in the workplace. That rash was a direct result from the stress of the situation. I immediately decided I needed to quit my job. After my last day of work I never experienced that rash again. I learned that we feed ourselves much more than merely food; our thoughts feed us as well.

Our thoughts either build us up or they deplete us. Our thoughts and emotions are either inflammatory or anti-inflammatory. Circumstances happen to us, but we give that event a meaning. We give that event an interpretation that either serves us, or disempowers us. We have power over our thoughts, we decide whether they are empowering or whether they deplete us. We possess the ability to create the health that we want and the health that we deserve. We also possess the ability to reverse or slow the aging process. Yes, it's true! You can look and feel younger!

I learned that food directly impacts not only our physical health, but also directly impacts our brain, mental health and emotions. If that were not enough, food impacts our consciousness. I began to notice that people I knew that had chosen to be vegans seemed to have a certain peace about them. There was something different about them.

I realized, after speaking with my vegan friends and family as well as researching the vegan lifestyle, that their diet was affecting their consciousness. Factory raised animals are treated in ways that would be considered a felony if you treated your pet that way. Not only that, when animals are slaughtered they smell death in the slaughterhouse. They hear the screams and squeals of pain and fear from the animals being slaughtered. They feel the terror. They experience the most extreme fear, knowing they are going to die. Hormones race through their bodies in response to their pending death. Their bodies vibrate panic and horror. Their death is a brutal, painful death.

When we purchase the meat at the grocery store, it is clean and neatly packaged. There is little evidence of the fear and brutality the animal suffered during its life and its death. However, when that piece of meat is consumed, we are eating all the hormones that were coursing through the animal's bodies before it was slaughtered; we are consuming all the fear and terror experienced by the animal. We are absorbing that consciousness.

Vegans do not consume those hormones; they do not consume the fear and terror. Their consciousness is not being adversely affected by their dietary choices.

If you choose to eat meat or dairy, I would like to suggest that you research how the animals are raised, fed, and treated throughout their lifetime, making sure that the animals are raised and slaughtered humanely. It takes time to take responsibility for what we consume. I encourage you to research the sources of your food so you can make wise food choices for you and your family. I believe the results will provide you with healthy rewards. If you choose to be an omnivore, I would like to recommend www.livestockconservancy.org to begin your research. The humane treatment of livestock benefits the animal, but also directly impacts your health and journey to enlightened, youthful living.

It is my desire that this book will inspire you to think about your health and the aging process in a different light. Maybe it will spark you to explore different lifestyle choices and design a lifestyle that truly serves you and works towards slowing or reversing the aging process. This book is designed to serve as a tool and a guide, helping you to achieve optimum health; a resource to help you reverse any chronic conditions you may be experiencing; and give you the extra edge you have been looking for in attaining a youthful, sexier body and mind - at any age.

This book will supply you with simple tips and easy steps to follow allowing you to upgrade and improve the level of your health and well-being based upon what you put in and on your body.

Lessons Learned

- Symptoms are our friends. They are our body's way to communicate to us.
- Your body has the ability to heal itself, given we remove the toxins and feed it the proper fuel.
- There is a direct connection between our dietary choices, thoughts and emotions and any physical symptoms we may be experiencing.

Exercise

Write out your health story. What health challenges have you faced over the years? What is your diet? Is there a common thread in your story?

Follow this link to download the 60-Day Anti-Aging Body Master Plan worksheet to help you track and create your personalized Master Plan. By writing out your thoughts and ideas, you will be designing your blueprint for success!

http://goo.gl/E5FFMj

CHAPTER THREE

Power of Food

---

*"Let your food be your medicine and let your medicine
be your food."*

Hippocrates

The power of food is extraordinary. To get a clear understanding of the difference between food, medicine and drugs as I view it, here are some definitions:

Drug - A substance taken for its narcotic or stimulant effects. All drugs impair or halt enzyme activity.

Medicine - The science of treating or preventing disease or other damage to the body, mind or spirit through diet, exercise and other nonsurgical means.

Food - A material usually of plant or animal origin that contains or consists of essential body nutrients and is ingested and assimilated by an organism, in order to maintain life and growth.

Food: Is It Anti-Aging Medicine or Is It a Drug?

For millennia food has been our medicine and medicine has been our food. You can clearly see this if you study indigenous cultures,

Ayurvedic traditions and Tradition Chinese Medicine. It has not been until fairly recently that we have introduced processed and artificial foods into our diets which function in the same manner as synthetic drugs. In our westernized culture, we have confused drugs with medicine, especially when it comes to food.

In our culture we are not using food intentionally. We tend to eat to quiet down and quell the physical pangs of hunger. We do not think about using food to foster health and vitality. We tend to think of food in terms of convenience. When it is breakfast time we make ourselves a bowl of oatmeal, or order bacon, eggs and hash browns, chasing it down with a cup of coffee with artificial creamer and artificial sweetener or orange juice from concentrate.

For lunch we eat a sandwich with potato chips. For dinner we get a plate of pasta or steak and potatoes. We tend to eat according to breakfast foods, lunch foods or dinner foods. We may snack on a piece of fruit or on a candy bar throughout the day. We try and eat healthfully, we read the labels, we make sure that the foods are low in fat, sodium or sugar; but our lives are busy and we tend to eat on the go, intending to make it up at the next meal - or do better tomorrow.

We eat in front of our computers and we eat in our cars. We do not have a ritual around our meals. Not much thought is being put into each meal with regard to its purpose. Why are you eating what you are eating? What impact will that food have on your body, on your mind or on your emotions?

I ran into a friend of mine in court recently. He knows my passion for food and healthy eating. He was walking down the hallway with chips and soda in his hand. He was excited to tell me that he was having a diet soda with his nacho cheese flavored chips. Since he was trying to lose a few pounds, he was proud of his choice of the diet soda, believing that it cancelled out the calories in the chips!

Going back to the idea of food as medicine, all food functions as medicine or as a drug. I differentiate between drugs, that are not life enhancing, and medicine which serves to enrich health and vitality. Drugs are toxic as in chemotherapy and medicine is restorative as in essential oils. There is a broad spectrum in between. Think about this, drugs, whether obtained via a prescription or over-the-counter, always carry risks. These substances always have side effects. The one advantage of taking a drug over eating processed foods is that you can read the product insert which details all the possible side effects. Unfortunately, there are no product inserts with chips, white bread or even the canned vegetable drink.

All drugs impact enzyme activity in the body. That is why we experience side effects. Enzymes are the spark of life. If we do not have enzyme activity we die. We cannot even blink an eye without enzymes.

If you eat fake food like cookies, pasta, donuts and other processed foods they have no nutritional value; they are devoid of enzymes. They act just like drugs in that they cause side effects. They cause us to get sugar highs; they cause us to get high triglycerides or diabetes, heart disease and even certain cancers. In short, they accelerate the aging process. We are eating ourselves old.

Processed foods cause mood disorders, leaky gut and can even lead to autoimmune diseases. We eat ourselves into these conditions then go to the doctor to get drugs to alleviate the symptoms. These "foods" come with a whole host of unwanted side effects. Many times people need another prescription to alleviate the side effects caused by the previous drug. We may resort to all sorts of extreme medical interventions to achieve the health and appearance that is our birthright.

How many people would be outraged if we knew drugs caused diseases or death? Look at the Vioxx debacle. People suffered and died, families were destroyed, lawsuits erupted and the product was ultimately taken off the market, after causing over 60,000 deaths. In fact, Merck, was even criminally prosecuted due to its actions. But no one bats an eye when people are suffering from diabetes or heart disease due to the "foods" they are eating.

If we become conscious about our food decisions and view food as medicine, which is healing and life-enhancing, then we can eat our way back to health, we can eat our way back off of the drugs and reverse the aging process.

Food Has a Direct Impact Behavior

Linus Pauling once stated, "The functioning of the brain is dependent on its composition and structure that is on the molecular environment." You are what you eat. Think about a high performance vehicle, a Ferrari for example. It is not designed to run on regular gasoline; it may run but will not perform optimally.

Once it starts pinging, sputtering, backfiring and having mechanical issues, you would not take it to the mechanic and ask for replacement parts and expect it to run as a finely tuned instrument if you are still giving it regular gasoline. If you do, the mechanic may change the filters on the car, he may change the spark plugs, and he may change any number of parts and tune the engine.

If he is able to finely tune the vehicle again so it is running smoothly and has that characteristic Ferrari sound and you continue to put the regular gasoline in, the same symptoms are going to come back. This is exactly what we do to our bodies. We feed ourselves crappy fuel that our bodies were not designed to run on. We feed ourselves processed flour, processed sugar, trans fats, artificial flavors and preservatives.

Then we wonder why we experience symptoms. We become lethargic; we get brain fog, acne, constipation, hot flashes. We go to the doctor because we do not like the symptoms and we walk away with a pill. The amazing thing is that the pill seems to work. It alleviated the symptom that we came in for, hallelujah!

The problem is we develop a new symptom and many times these new symptoms are silently developing within us. We do not even realize it is there until one day we develop another condition like heart disease. We have been conditioned to think to ourselves that "it is just old age catching up to me," or "I am falling apart."

In reality, the problem is the fuel we feed ourselves. We are the finely tuned Ferrari trying to function on cheap, leaded gasoline. Have you ever heard of the Twinkie defense? Dan White was standing trial for the murders of Harvey Milk who was a San Francisco City Supervisor, and George Mosconi, the Mayor of San Francisco. White's attorney claimed that he was suffering from depression as a consequence of changing his diet from healthy food to sugary junk foods. The argument was that he was suffering from depression due to his diet. In turn, the depression caused him to suffer from diminished capacity which is when he committed the murders.

We all know that drugs are powerful. That is why we need a prescription for so many of them. They are carefully formulated to boost our moods, reduce our cholesterol or alleviate pain. Don't be deceived. All drugs come with a long list of side effects, usually in such fine print that nobody reads them. In our fast paced society we want that instant gratification. We want that symptom to go away - NOW!

Foods are powerful, too. They can impact us just like drugs. Foods, especially fake foods have the ability to influence our bodies and our minds just like drugs. The only difference is that "foods" don't come with an insert of fine print describing its side effects. When I talk about fake "foods" I am talking about things like aspartame, Splenda, trans fats, and margarine. Any kind of processed foods (such as flour, pastries, and chips), excitotoxins like MSG, neurotoxins, natural flavorings are all fake, manufactured "foods." The reality is, they are not foods at all. They are drugs.

You are going to find most of these "food" products were touted as the latest and greatest health food. The sugar substitutes are promoted by the food industry as a great substitute to having sugar in your diet. It turns out we are all part of a human experiment. It is not until years later that research proves that these substances are so dangerous to us that they cause illness and disease.

Look at what happened with saccharin. Saccharin was a "great" sugar substitute and was being promoted heavily. Then it turned out that it was carcinogenic. People were trying to save 15 calories from a sugar packet over 0 calories in a saccharine. Really? Is saving that 15 calories worth exposing yourself to cancer.

Look at trans fats, which are fake fats. This is another product that was promoted as the latest and greatest diet food; it was intended to be the cure all for heart disease, for fat loss and ending weight gain. It turns out that this is one of the most dangerous "foods" that there is and is currently being taken off the market.

Then there are MSG and other excitotoxins. These chemicals excite the cells so much that they open up and they allow too much calcium in, causing nerve damage and ultimately cell death.

Natural flavorings present more health issues. We think that natural flavors, for example natural strawberry flavor comes from strawberries. Nothing can be further from the truth. There was a recent 20/20 expose` called The Flavorist. It talked about the science behind these food companies who are developing flavors.

Natural flavorings can actually come from the anal gland of the beaver. What they do is excrete a substance called castoreum from castor sacs near the anal gland and use it to create "natural" flavors. It is pretty disgusting! But they can call it natural because it comes from the beaver. So now days any time I look at something that says natural flavors, I think of the beaver butt and I put it back on the shelf.

This "natural" flavor is the substance that is used in many processed foods, candies and beverages. Typically it is listed as vanilla, strawberry or raspberry flavoring. The FDA has deemed it GRAS, which stands for Generally Regarded as Safe.

Foods these days are addictive just like drugs are addictive. The food companies employ scientist to make foods taste good and to make them addictive so they sell more. There are major R & D departments that do research on how much salt a food should contain, how much sugar a food should contain and how much fat a food should contain.

Watch television commercials and see the manner in which foods are being promoted. For example, if a "food" is promoted as low in sodium it will usually be high in sugar or fat to ensure that it is tasty. Low fat foods tend to have higher sugar content.

These companies are masters at manipulating the recipes, playing around with the salt, sugar and fat content in order to make them more addictive. Then they add potent flavorings and other enchantments like MSG ensuring these foods taste good and are addictive. When you bite into the product you get a powerful burst of flavor. That powerful burst of flavor cannot compare to the flavor of biting into a fresh strawberry or an orange.

Billions of dollars are being spent each year by these food companies to engineer "foods" to taste good and make them more addictive. Always, the end result is increased sales. When formulating these "foods" there is little to no concern for your health or the health of your children. In fact, these companies know exactly what they are doing. The objective in designing "foods" such as Lucky Charms and pop tarts is to make them bright and colorful, bursting with flavor, directly targeting our children.

One of the things that really interests me about food and the power of food is the impact that it has upon our behaviors and our thought processes. I became fascinated in this with regard to my clients. As a criminal defense attorney a lot of my clients have addiction issues and behavioral issues. They don't think through the decisions they are making. They are impulsive.

What I have done in my practice is talked with my clients about their food and food choices. I discover what they are eating. What I find is that most of them are consuming most of their meals at fast food restaurants, drinking a lot of soda, eating a lot of chips and processed foods and their food choices do impact their behavior. I read a book by Barbara Stitt; she is an amazing woman who was a probation officer in Minneapolis many years ago.

She made the link between food and behavior. She had suffered from hypoglycemia herself. Her hypoglycemia symptoms were so profound that it startled and scared her. She started doing research and discovered the impact that her diet had upon her mental and emotional states. Changing her diet had such a profound impact upon her that she started educating her probationers. When they implemented her advice and adhered to pure whole food diet eliminating soda and processed foods, the recidivism rate decreased sharply.

In her jurisdiction young, juvenile probationers for the most part would reoffend 80% to 90% of the time. However after following her dietary advice, those statistics were flipped; about 80% to 90% of her probationers never reoffended again. If they would go off of the whole food diet and start drinking soda and eating the chips and sugared cereals they would start to experience the impulsivity, hostility, aggression and other emotions that had gotten them into trouble in the first place. Food is extremely, extremely powerful, and unfortunately overlooked.

Another example of the power of food comes out of a prison in San Bernardino, California. In the late 1990's the prison instituted a program, allowing the prisoners to opt whether to be housed on the side of the prison that served a conventional prison diet or to be housed on the side of the prison that served a vegan diet.

The results were stunning. Remarkable behavioral changes were observed in the prison yard. The prison officials noted that they did not encounter the usual racial disputes. Nobody "owned" or controlled the yard. Everyone played basketball together. The typical racial lines were not drawn between gang member, Blacks and Hispanics. The other side of the prison which served the conventional prison diet experienced the same racial divisions and problems that were present at any other prison.

Remarkably the vegan inmates described having greater energy, increased stamina and reduced problems with acne.

Fake foods are powerful; and if fake foods can impact our bodies and our emotions and our lives to such a degree that it influences criminal behavior, what impact do whole pure foods make on our lives? They have the power to lift our mood and the vibrational energy to heal. They have the power to keep our minds sharp, well into our senior years. Alzheimer's disease and dementia are not a normal, inevitable result of aging - even though they are now common results of aging.

The question to ask yourself is how will you use food? As a medicine or as a drug?

Foods Possess Vibrational, Healing Energy

The sun provides life force for all living beings and plants. Life would not exist without the sun. Its benefits are extensive. Sun exposure causes our bodies to synthesis vitamin D. It helps regulate the circadian rhythms allowing us to sleep and to regenerate.

Consider a plant. The sun's life force is synthesized by the plant, making chlorophyll. Plants are made up of the high vibrational, life-giving energy of the sun. When we eat produce we are consuming this healing life force. The foods that have absorbed and transmuted this energy of the sun possess the highest nutrient value known.

Look at chlorophyll; it is one molecule different than blood. The center atom in blood is iron, while the center atom in chlorophyll is magnesium. Chlorophyll is the blood and the life force of the plant just as the blood in our bodies is our life force. If our blood is healthy and clean, our bodies are going to be healthy and clean. Chlorophyll is extremely nutrient dense and is very cleansing to our bodies. It is a blood cleanser as well as a blood builder.

This is one of the substances that my chiropractor put me on when I was suffering with my intestinal issues. I directly attribute my healing to the cleansing power of chlorophyll.

There are many high vibration foods. These include the super foods. Super foods are foods that have high mineral content, high vitamin content and the life force energy from the sun.

Researcher, Bruce Tainio, has analyzed and calibrated the frequency of many different substances, including the frequency of foods, frequency of the human body, and even the frequencies at which people get sick. He discovered the average frequency of the human body during the daytime is 62 to 68 hertz.

The healthy body frequency is 62 to 72 hertz. When the frequency drops the immune system is compromised. Amazingly, he has been able to calibrate the frequency of different body parts. The genius brain calibrated at a frequency of 80 to 82 megahertz. The brain frequency calibrated at 72 to 90 megahertz. A normal brain frequency is 72 megahertz.

Considering this, it makes sense to incorporate high vibration foods into your diet to raise the vibrational frequency of our brains. In calibrating foods, it was discovered that fresh organic foods vibrate at a higher frequency than the conventionally grown foods. Fresh foods vibrate at the rate of 20 to 27 hertz; same with herbs. Dried foods are lower, from 15 to 22 hertz; the same with dried herbs.

Processed and canned foods calibrated at 0 hertz. Looking at the state of our society and culture, it is no surprise that our diets consist predominately of processed, packaged foods.

Doctor and researcher, Dr. David Hawkins, has a huge body of work in which he has calibrated emotions as well as other substances. According to Dr. Hawkins synthetics, plastics, artificial coloring, preservatives, insecticides, artificial sweeteners all weaken us, which is no surprise when you think about it. He has also determined that pure organic substances strengthen us. Again it makes sense to feed our bodies pure organic substances.

The highest vibration foods are the ones that deeply absorb the life force of the sun. Wheat grass, phytoplankton and chlorophyll are the highest vibration foods known. Super foods such as raw cacao, seaweed, spirulina and goji berries all possess extremely high life force from the sun, as well as a high mineral content. They are nutrient dense, life enhancing, anti-aging foods.

Root vegetables such as potatoes, sweet potatoes and beets are grown under the earth and are unable to directly absorb the life energy of the sun. Because they possess lower vibrational energy, I recommend these foods not be the mainstay of your diet.

Things like eggs, cheese and dairy, do not possess the sun's life force energy. Therefore they vibrate at a very low degree if they vibrate at all.

Albert Einstein said, "Everything is energy and that is all there is to it. Match the frequency of the reality you want and you cannot help but to get that reality. It can be no other way. This is not philosophy, this physics".

Bruce Tainio, as I mentioned, calibrated the frequency in which people get disease and illness. Colds and flus start at 57 to 60 megahertz; disease starts at 58 megahertz. Candida overgrowth starts 55 megahertz and people are receptive to cancer at 42 megahertz. Death begins at 25 megahertz.

What reality do you want to create? A high vibrational, vital life? A lifestyle that reverses aging? Then, I suggest incorporating high vibrational foods into every meal.

Vibration of Emotion Can Heal or Cause Disease

Dr. David Hawkins wrote a book entitled Power verses Force. In that book he detailed how he was able to calibrate emotions. Interestingly, enlightenment calibrated at the highest vibration. Emotions play a critical role in our overall health as illustrated by Dr. Hawkins' extensive research.

Level	Emotion	Scale	Process	Life View	
Enlightenment, Various levels	Ineffable	700-1000	Pure Consciousness	Is	**POWER**
Peace	Bliss	600	Illumination	Perfect	
Joy	Serenity	540	Transfiguration	Complete	
Love (Unconditional)	Reverence	500	Revelation	Benign	
Reason	Understanding	400	Abstraction	Meaningful	
Acceptance	Forgiveness	350	Transcendence	Harmonious	
Willingness	Optimism	310	Intention	Hopeful	
Neutrality	Trust	250	Release	Satisfactory	
Courage	Affirmation	200	Empowerment	Feasible	
Pride	Scorn	175	Inflation	Demanding	**FORCE**
Anger	Hate	150	Aggression	Antagonistic	
Desire	Craving	125	Enslavement	Disappointing	
Fear	Anxiety	100	Withdrawal	Frightening	
Grief	Regret	75	Despondency	Tragic	
Apathy	Despair	50	Abdication	Hopeless	
Guilt	Blame	30	Destruction	Condemnation	
Shame	Humiliation	20	Elimination	Miserable	

This chart explains why it is so important to prepare and eat your foods with love and gratitude. One of my favorite restaurants, Café Gratitude, names each of its dishes not for the ingredients but for the intention for the food. For example, one of the dishes is called "I am Grateful." When you receive your dish the server places it in front of you and says, "You are Grateful." What a beautiful way to start your dining experience.

Based upon what we learned from Albert Einstein, Dr. Hawkins and Bruce Tainio, to name a few, it is imperative to employ all means available to raise our vibrational energy in order to realize the level of health, youthfulness, beauty and enlightenment that we deserve and that has been eluding you.

Lessons Learned

- Food can function as medicine to help you heal
- Food can function as a drug and cause unwanted side effects
- Food has a direct impact upon your behavior, emotions and clarity of your mind

Action Steps

- Don't eat merely to fill up your stomach. Choose foods based upon their function and how they will make you feel.
- Research drugs you are currently taking and try to find foods/supplements that can address your symptoms without any of the unwanted side effects.

Exercise

For 1 week, record the following: Every food and beverage that crosses your lips; The emotions you experience throughout the day.

List all medications you take, whether prescription or over-the-counter medication.

CHAPTER FOUR

Anti-Aging Body Strategies - The Detox Lifestyle

"The ultimate cause of human disease is the consequence of our transgression of the universal laws of life."

Paracelsus

Detoxing Slows the Aging Process

We get toxins from our food, from the air we breathe and from our environment. Toxins are inhaled, ingested and absorbed through our skin. Toxins are everywhere in the environment; we get them from pollution, from our body care products and even our thoughts and emotions can be toxic. It is over time that our body gets overwhelmed as the toxins accumulate.

If our bodies cannot eliminate the toxins we are exposed to on a daily basis, we are designed with a back-up plan. The number one priority of the body is to keep us alive and protect our vital organs at all cost. Part of our body's back-up plan is to escort the toxins away from the vital organs and store them in the fat cells. Consider this, if you are unable to lose weight, one reason might be that your body is overwhelmed by toxins. If you lose the excess fat, the toxins may have nowhere to go. Your body may actually be protecting you from the toxins. Excess fat can be a protective mechanism.

But it's not necessarily as simple as that. Not all toxins are stored in fat cells. They circulate through the body, causing wear and tear on your organs, digestive system, immune system, circulatory system, wreaking havoc on whatever is the weakest body system or organ.

Degenerative diseases can develop as a result of a toxic body. Even though our bodies are resilient they are constantly assaulted by toxins. When the toxins build up over time, our bodies get overwhelmed, symptoms begin to appear and then eventually, with the passage of time degenerative diseases begin to set in. It all begins with the toxic build up.

But where do these toxins come from? Most of us try to live a clean, healthy life. However, you might be surprised to find out several common sources of toxins. They come from all different places and come at us from all different directions. We get them from the foods we eat, from the body care products we use, and even as a byproduct from our thoughts and emotions. Toxins cannot be avoided and are a part of our everyday lives. Since we cannot entirely eliminate them, it is imperative to develop a detox lifestyle.

We produce toxic waste from the normal metabolic processes occurring within our bodies every moment of every day. Take a look at each individual cell. What does each and every one of them need? All of them, without exception, need three things: oxygen, nutrients and the ability to excrete the metabolic waste. Each cell, each organ, and our bodies as a whole all need these three things in order to survive and thrive.

Nobel Prize winner, Dr. Alexis Carrel, developed keen interest blood transfusion and organ transplantation. He pioneered efforts to maintain tissue cultures. He developed the art of keeping cells and tissues alive in the laboratory. One of his experiments involved taking the tissue from the heart of a chicken embryo and keeping it alive for over 34 years! The tissue was kept alive because each individual cell was given what it needed: oxygen, the right nutrients, and a clean living environment. Carrel had designed a system where he was able to make sure the cells were provided a consistent supply of oxygen and nutrients. On top of that, he insured the cells were not poisoned by their own metabolic waste.

In fact, these cells outlived him. The experiment was deliberately terminated after Carrel had passed away.

Inflammation and Oxidation - Root Causes of Accelerated Aging

We hear a lot about inflammation and oxidation these days. We hear how detrimental they are to our health. However, that is not necessarily the case. It is <u>chronic</u> inflammation and <u>chronic</u> oxidation that are detrimental to our health.

In fact, inflammation is critical to maintaining your health. I know that may sound like a foreign concept because we are taught how damaging inflammation is to our bodies. But acute inflammation is a normal, healthy response to injury or infection. It is your body's attempt to protect itself and remove the harmful stimuli.

If you are doing some work around the house and you stub your toe, it will bleed, get red and inflamed and that is all good; that is the normal healing process. Your body is trying to make sure no infection sets in and is working to heal and repair the damaged tissue. Reaching for a non-steroidal anti-inflammatory drug (NSAID) like ibuprofen will not serve you. It might make you feel better in the moment, but it will prolong the healing time. It will only interfere with the natural healing process of the body.

With more than 30 billion doses of NSAIDs consumed annually in the United States alone, it is important to look at the risks these drugs pose. There are significant side effects to taking NSAIDs. In addition to them destroying vitamin C (which is a powerful antioxidant) and slowing fracture healing, NSAIDs common side effects include inflammatory bowel disease, leaky gut, hemorrhaging in your gastrointestinal tract, erectile dysfunction, liver damage, renal failure, heart attack and stroke. They may help to temporarily ease the pain, but they prolong the healing time. I think it is important to ask yourself whether they worth the risk?

Most people do not realize this, but over-the-counter pain relievers are some of the deadliest drugs out there. Every year over one hundred thousand people are hospitalized with serious side effects from taking NSAIDs.

More than four times as many people die from NSAID side effects than from cervical cancer each year. That is absolutely crazy! This is stuff that doctors are promoting. One of the scariest things about these drugs is that only one in five people that develop serious problems have had any early warning symptoms.

Chronic Inflammation Causes Chronic Age Related Conditions

It is only when the inflammation gets out of control, when it becomes chronic, that it can become deadly! So, how do we tame the inflammation beast? By uncovering the root of the problem: chronic inflammation which occurs when there is cellular stress. What causes the cellular stress? Lack of proper nutrients, lack of adequate oxygen, and when the cells are swimming in their own metabolic waste are the common causes of cellular stress.

The typical Standard American Diet (SAD) is an inflammatory diet. Consuming grains, breads, pasta, refined sugar - just about all simple carbohydrates - have a high glycemic index and cause blood sugar to rise quickly. This causes a cascade effect releasing pro-inflammatory hormones.

If eating simple carbohydrates weren't bad enough, combining them with polyunsaturated vegetable oils (PUFAs) like safflower, corn, sunflower, soy, peanut and vegetable oil, are disastrous! The inflammatory effects of these foods erode the integrity of the cells, the organs and the entire body.

Inflammatory conditions can be life threatening. The damage is being done silently, over time. You may begin to notice random symptoms. There doesn't seem to be a link between these symptoms at first. And, they are routinely dismissed as "old age." Ultimately, the doctor declares his diagnosis: asthma, rheumatoid arthritis, heart disease, diabetes, diverticulitis, Crohn's disease, Alzheimer's disease, gingivitis, some cancers, or even depression. The uncontrolled chronic inflammation can, and does, affect each and every tissue of the body.

And NSAIDs don't help with chronic inflammation, despite their name. As discussed earlier, they may get rid of the acute symptom, but they simultaneously induce chronic inflammation.

When you begin to address these chronic inflammatory conditions, I recommend taking a step back and examining what caused the so-called dis-ease. What caused the inflammation in the first place?

The first step is to assess where you are; taking a good, hard look at your lifestyle. Recognize that you have the power to influence your chronic inflammatory response. Have you adopted a pro-inflammatory lifestyle? Do you drink plenty of fresh water? It is a good idea to get in the habit of drinking half your weight in ounces every day. Are you eating a healthy diet? Foods that are rich in antioxidants? Are you enjoying foods rich in essential fatty acids on a daily basis?

For optimal health and longevity, you will be well served by eating lots of fresh, organic, non-starchy vegetables; eliminating sugar and processed foods; supplementing with vitamins and minerals; exercising; and meditating on a daily basis. Take time for yourself to de-stress. These are all things that are going to help your body to heal from chronic inflammation.

Chronic Oxidation Depletes Anti-Aging Nutrients

When we are looking at inflammation you also have to look at oxidation. Oxidation and inflammation are two conditions that are pretty much joined at the hip with each other; you cannot have one without the other. So, what is oxidation? When it is under control, it is a normal, healthy metabolic process. It is a process where energy is created at the cellular level. And we all want energy, don't we?

When oxidation is rampant, it damages the body. The simplest analogy is that of rust. When a nail is exposed to the elements, it rusts. If the nail is protected, it does not rust. In our bodies, oxidative stress results in free-radical damage. It is the oxidative stress that is dangerous to our health and must be kept under control

Again, we cannot just get rid of oxidation. It is essential for the digestive process; it breaks down nutrients, it helps improve metabolism and it increases the production of energy. It is used by the immune system as a way to attack and kill pathogens. It is not the oxidation itself that is bad; it is the out-of-control oxidation that is detrimental because that is what causes free radical damage.

Free radical damage, just like chronic inflammation is largely lifestyle dependent. Cigarette smoke, pollution, pesticides on our foods and alcohol all trigger free radical damage. Free radicals can damage the DNA, causing the cell to mutate. The end result can lead to chronic diseases, accelerated aging, Parkinson's disease, heart failure, Alzheimer's disease, cancer and Chronic Fatigue Syndrome.

A huge step to arresting the free radical damage and reverse chronic conditions is to detoxify the body and give ourselves the nutrients that we need.

Antioxidants are critical component to help the body detox. Antioxidants include Vitamins A, C, E and selenium. Great sources of antioxidants include blueberries, goji berries, raw cacao and blue-green algae.

Proper Digestion is the Key to an Anti-Aging Body

It is my belief that almost every chronic health condition that plagues our society is acquired through lifestyle choices. For now, lets focus on our daily food choices, which can lead to either the liver being overwhelmed or the digestion not functioning properly. Digestion is key to our health. Not one step of the digestive process can be ignored.

Let me give you a very quick overview of the digestive process. Chewing each bite of your meal breaks it down mechanically as well as causing it to be thoroughly coated with saliva, which is rich in amylase, helping to break it down enzymatically. When the food hits the stomach, stomach acid and more enzymes are released, breaking down protein; as the contents leave the stomach, and enters the duodenum bile is excreted to allow for the digestion and utilization of fats. As your meal travels through the small intestine, it is being further digested. The nutrients are absorbed by the villi in the small intestine. Digestion includes the entire process from what goes into the mouth to what comes out the other end. It is important to pay particular attention to the gut.

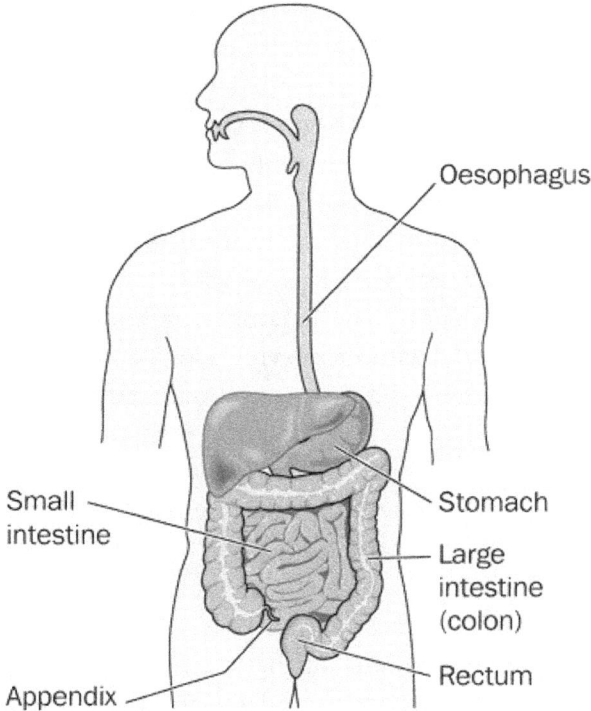

The gut is known as the second brain - some scientists even refer to it as the first brain! We all are aware of the importance of our brain. Great care is taken in protecting it. There are helmet laws on the books; there are EEGs to measure the electrical activity of the brain; there are nutrients essential to the health of the brain. No one would dispute the significance of the brain.

Considering the gut is called the second brain, the same care and attention should be paid to it. I would like to point out two important facts about the gut. First, about 80% of the immune system is in the gut; and second, over 80% of the serotonin is found in the gut, not the brain!

The importance of healthy digestion cannot be underestimated. It is important to me to educate my clients on the importance of the digestive process and of their food choices. I explain that to achieve optimal health, the foods they put in their bodies must be of the best quality possible because, when broken down, these foods become the building blocks of our bodies. The nutrients from our foods are the building blocks of our organs, of our brain, and of each and every one of our cells. But this is only part of the battle. Consider this: If we are not able to break down those foods, even if we eat the best protein, fats, and carbohydrates, we will run into two issues.

One, we won't be able to assimilate and get the benefit of those nutrients. Two, we are not able to eliminate the waste; if you are not able to eliminate the waste your body is going to become toxic. Toxins are going to be circulating throughout your body. These two tasks cannot be accomplished without enzyme activity.

Enzymes are indispensable to digestion. Enzymes are the spark of life; nothing can happen in your body without them. You cannot blink an eye without enzyme activity. The analogy I like to use is that of building a house. Let's say you have an empty lot, which represents your body. And, you have a master plan.

You order all the building supplies; you have the lumber, concrete, windows, nails and all the raw materials to build the house. They are delivered and they are put on the lot. The raw materials are like the carbs, fats, protein, vitamins and the minerals. You have all the materials on the lot.

If you do not have the workers, all of those materials are going to be sitting on the lot exposed to the elements and they are going to rot and deteriorate. Enzymes are the workers; nothing can get done without the enzymes. They are what break apart the nutrients so your body can absorb them. Optimal enzyme activity is critical to our health.

Enzymes become depleted if our bodies get overwhelmed with poor food choices, excess food, negative emotions, or stress. About 10% of our body's energy is used digesting and assimilating nutrients from our foods. I believe it is fundamental to optimal health to take digestive enzymes whenever you eat. This helps to take some of the strain off of the body which in turn will allow more energy to be available to focus other metabolic activities; ultimately, increasing our health and vitality.

Enzymes are used in the entire digestive and assimilation process so when you eat that beautiful fresh salad your body is able to fully utilize the nutrients that you are consuming.

They are found in all living plants and fruits. That is why it is of upmost importance to eat fresh pure foods. I recommend that a majority of your diet consist of fresh, organic, uncooked fruits and vegetables. Cooking plant based food over 105 to 118 degrees Fahrenheit kills their enzymes, leaving the food devoid of enzyme activity. If the food is devoid of enzyme activity, an added burden will be placed on your body.

I focus on having a diet rich in fresh, organic uncooked vegetables and fruits. Personally, I incorporate a lot of organic salads with fresh spinach, baby greens, tomatoes, and sprouts in my diet. Sprouts are awesome for an added boost of enzyme activity.

I also like to use bell pepper, cucumber, avocado, tomatoes, cilantro and onion to make a beautiful fresh salad. Fresh fruit such as apples, grapes, watermelon, and cantaloupe are also great additions to your salad, making them tasty and interesting.

Have you ever seen an apple on the ground that has fallen from the tree? If you pick up the apple you will see that it has a bruise on it, a spot that is brown and mushy. That bruise is the result of enzyme activity that is breaking down the apple. When we consume supplemental enzymes or foods that are rich in enzymes our meal is being broken down so that our bodies can utilize the nutrients in the food. It is supposed to break down that way. This is normal and healthy.

I had heard of an experiment that was done and wanted to actually see it for myself. I went and bought a kid's meal at McDonalds. I bought this meal over two years ago and I still have that meal today. It is sitting in the same paper bag that they served it to me in. The hamburger looks as beautiful as it did two years ago. There is no mold, it does not stink. In fact, it smells the same as it did 2 years ago; it is not being broken down at all. The French fries look the same as they did two years ago. You can put this "meal" on a plate and it looks the same as it did two years ago. The only difference between this "meal" and a "fresh" Happy Meal is the one I have is hard.

If you are eating these "foods" as a regular part of your diet, your body is not going to be able to break them down and it will be difficult to eliminate them. There are no nutrients for your body to assimilate.

This "food" is just sitting inside your gut, not being digested and utilized by your body. This is no way to treat your second brain!

It is important to determine if we are unnecessarily creating toxicity in our bodies. Toxicity comes from a variety of sources, not just from dietary sources. Toxicity comes from pollution, body care products, cleaning products, food additives. The list is seemingly endless! No matter the source of the toxicity, it creates an unhealthy burden, which ultimately will result in unwanted symptoms. There is a broad range of symptoms from headaches, allergies, skin issues, to diabetes, and more. Review the list that follows to determine the level of toxins in your life.

Are you toxic?

Do you have sugar cravings?
Do you drink alcohol?
Do you eat processed foods?
Do you bathe, wash your hair or hands with ingredients you cannot pronounce?
Do you use lotion that contain ingredients you cannot pronounce?
Do you use anti-bacterial soaps or lotions?
Do you use make-up that is not organic?
Do you use sunscreen?
Do you use antiperspirant?
Do you have dental work such as amalgam fillings?
Do you have retainers or other dental work with metal?
Do you have root canals?
Do you have dental implants?
Do you use toothpaste with fluoride?
Do you use toothpaste with glycerine?
Do you use tap water to drink?
Do you use tap water to shower?
Do you smoke?
Are you around people who smoke?
Do you dye your hair?
Do you use nail polish?

Do you have acrylic nails?

Do you take prescription medication?

Do you take over-the-counter medication?

Do you use cologne or perfume?

Do you have chronic headaches?

Do you suffer from arthritis?

Do you have frequent illnesses?

Do you suffer from unexplained aches and pains?

Do you have sensitivity to perfumes?

Do you have sensitivity to smoke?

Do you have chronic infections?

Do you suffer hair loss?

Do you suffer from flushing or hot flashes?

Do you experience bloating?

Do you have a history of belching or passing gas?

Do you experience hay fever or allergies?

Do you experience excessive weight gain?

Are you a compulsive eater?

Do you suffer from insomnia?

Do you have learning disabilities?

Do you suffer from anxiety or fear?

Are you angry or irritable?

Do you suffer from depression?

Do you suffer from fatigue?

Do you engage in destructive self-talk?

Do you experience mood swings?

If you answered "yes" to any of these questions, you may be toxic.

Turn Back the Hands of Time with Anti-Aging Cleansing Programs

There are several cleansing programs to help turn the tide in your favor on the inflammation and free radical damage. You can refer to my website www.Anti-AgingBody.com for details on these programs.

However, I would like to point out a few tips that will make any cleansing protocol more effective. First, drink plenty of water when you are on a cleanse. Second, make sure you are able to take it easy and really allow your body the time to relax and release the toxins it has been holding onto for so long. Third, get plenty of fresh air and sunshine during the cleansing period. And, finally, it is a great idea to incorporate dry-skin brushing and far-infrared saunas in your daily routine. It would be great to integrate these tips into your new Anti-Aging Body lifestyle that you are developing.

The Hormone Balancing Detox Diet

A cleansing program is something that is temporary, it is short term. This is not a lifestyle. But in order to maintain more detox oriented diet it is important to look and see what our bodies need in order to detox. When designing a detox diet it is fundamental to look at the organs of detoxification. One of the main organs of detoxification is the liver.

The liver is like a factory and it performs over 500 vital functions. Some of those functions include producing cholesterol, clearing blood of drugs and other poisonous or toxic substances and regulating blood clotting. The broken down toxic substances are ultimately excreted through the bowel or the urine. Considering all of these functions, it is no surprise that the liver needs specific nutrients in order function at its best and to detoxify your body.

Hormones play an integral role in the aging process. Since the subject of hormones is extremely complex, I will briefly touch on that topic here. The liver regulates, metabolizes and breaks down hormones such as estrogen, allowing excess hormones to be excreted from the body safely. The body's ability or lack there of to metabolize estrone, for example, is linked to estrogen-related cancers.

I have found that women have found significant relief from their menopausal symptoms by adhering to a liver detox lifestyle. Katie, a woman in her 50s was experiencing weight gain and daily hot flashes. I coached her through a liver flush and recommended a liver detox diet. After being on the program for 30 days, her hot flashes subsided and her weight normalized. I have discovered that following the protocols in the Anti-Aging Body has led to an easy transition for women going through menopause. In fact, I have clients that come to me to do a cleanse in order to relieve themselves of hot flashes.

The liver needs a broad array of antioxidants and their co-factors. Antioxidants help combat free radical damage. Antioxidants are found in the rich, colorful, deeply pigmented fruits and vegetables. Some examples of antioxidant rich foods are bell peppers that have the beautiful deep red, yellow and orange colors; pomegranates that have that gorgeous red color; blueberries, raspberries, blackberries, which possess intense purple, blue and red color.

In addition to antioxidants, the liver also uses methyl groups and sulfur to detoxify. You may be wondering what the heck are methyl groups and where are they found? Think about cruciferous vegetables. The cruciferous vegetables are vegetables that belong to the mustard family, such as broccoli, kale, cauliflower, mustard greens and cabbage. Sulfur containing foods include onions and garlic. When you are designing your detox diet these are the types of foods that I suggest incorporating on a regular basis to give yourself that extra edge. Give your organs the nutrients they need in order to be nourished and detoxify themselves.

Detoxing Emotions for Youthfulness

Any detoxification program would not be complete if we stopped at just the physical level. It is imperative to also look at detoxing ourselves emotionally. I believe that to achieve a state of true health, one must address their emotional wellbeing. There is a direct link between physical and emotional health. We all know that stress is a killer. It does not matter the source of the stress: physical, nutritional or emotional. When one is suffering from depression, panic attacks, anxiety, anger or frustration, they are ultimately experiencing stress.

Stress causes the body to release cortisol. Cortisol puts our bodies into the "fight or flight" mode. While in that mode, several things happen. Our immune system is suppressed and blood pressure is increased. The increased cortisol leads to decreased bone formation, leading to osteoporosis; cortisol causes collagen loss in the skin, leading to accelerated aging; and cortisol leads to muscle wasting, due to the cortisol prohibiting protein synthesis. There is not one part of the body that is spared the effects of stress! In fact, the first thing to shut down when we are stressed is our digestive system. It is ironic that many of us resort to eating when we are stressed, putting more of a burden on our gut.

Let's face it. We all want to look good. We want to look younger and turn back the hands of time. We don't want sagging skin or flabby muscles. It is time to do ourselves a favor, detox our lives by decreasing the stress in our lives. Our lives are dependent upon it. In fact, decreasing the stress in your life is one of the best anti-aging gifts you can give yourself.

One of the first places to start is to look at your self-talk. What do you say to yourself? Are you critical of your appearance? Do you beat yourself up when you make a mistake? Do you curse at yourself, call yourself stupid if you mess up?

Or do you treat yourself with compassion, the same compassion you would treat a friend or child if they made a mistake? We need to treat ourselves with compassion and grace in our inner dialogue.

Another great thing to do when detoxing emotions is to go on a fast - a gossip fast. Just commit to yourself that you are not going to gossip about people. If you cannot say something to somebody's face then you should not say it behind their back.

It's not enough to just stop beating ourselves up. We need to take it a step further and love and appreciate ourselves. The best way to do this is to create affirmations that acknowledge your talents, your strengths, and your beauty. Dare to acknowledge the best parts of you - and let them shine.

If you are struggling with self-talk, if you are struggling with beating yourself up, repeat to yourself affirmations in the morning and throughout the day. Post the affirmation on your mirror in the bathroom. Post it on your computer; post it in places where you will see it throughout the day. Give yourself affirmations about how smart you are, how capable you are, how worthy you are.

Another tip I use to help de-stress and detox negative emotions is to just take time to breathe deeply. When I take the time to breathe deeply and refocus my mind on the things I am grateful for, I become centered. I have an ever-growing list of things I am grateful for: my kids, my work, my clients, my assistant, my friends, the experiences I have had in my life that have led me to this place, my home. One of the most powerful habits you can develop is to focus on gratitude. Every morning upon waking up and every evening before drifting off to sleep, focus on the things that you are grateful for. Start your gratitude journal today. What are you grateful for?

I find it important to seek out experiences and employ a variety of strategies to manage the stressors in my life. I find it extremely valuable to make time to spend in nature. I live about 20 minutes from the beach, so when I feel especially disconnected, I will make the time to go to the beach and walk barefoot in the sand. I will also reset by going to a sensory deprivation tank. It is a two hour session where my senses are not bombarded by anything. I find it to be a completely rejuvenating experience! My de-stress tools in my tool box include meditation, yoga, deep breathing exercises and playing a musical instrument - even though I am not musically inclined!

And, as the saying goes, "Laughter is the best medicine." Watch a comedy, connect with a friend, do anything that brings you joy.

Creating Your Ideal Anti-Aging Environment

I would be remiss if I did not address your physical environment. I think that we underestimate the power of our physical environment. I ask myself these questions: What does my environment look like? What sounds are present? Can I incorporate beautiful scents into my space? Since this is where we live our lives, spending so much time in our homes, in our cars and at work, it is important to create sacred space. There is no doubt our environments impact us. I know that when my home is cluttered, if there are dirty dishes in the sink, I can't fully relax. I also know that when I surround myself with beauty whether it is from a picture, a screensaver on my computer, or just cleaning out my workspace I am able to relax.

Don't stop at creating a visually appealing environment. Go a step further and think about what sounds calm you. Do you like the sounds of nature or water? Maybe place a fountain near you? Is there background music that you can play? When you are choosing your music, pay attention to the words. Are they violent? Or is it music that soothes and fills your heart and soul?

Studies have shown that the sense of smell is the most powerful of all. To this day, if I smell "Cashmere Bouquet" soap, immediately I am transported back in time to my grandmother's house. I am reminded of the love I feel for her and of our special times together. You can use essential oils in a diffuser or nebulizer. Different scents can evoke different emotions. Jasmine can evoke the emotion of joy. Evergreen can take you back to Christmas. Do you have a favorite dish you can put on the stove that smells delicious and warms your heart?

Think of all the senses that you have - sight, smell, hearing, taste and touch. I recommend removing anything that does not serve you and create an environment that is as beautiful as you possibly can make it.

An Additional Note on Your Anti-Aging Environment

When you are creating your sacred space, consider what you are using to create the beauty. You don't want to remodel a room, for example, and find out that the new carpet is off-gassing and poisoning you and your family. Take the following test and see how non-toxic your environment is.

Is Your Home Toxic?

Could you eat off your floor after cleaning it with your favorite floor cleaner?
Can you safely wash out your mouth with your current soap?
Do any of the bottles under your sink contain anything that would send you to the Emergency Room if you drank it?
Is there any item under your sink that you would be able to water your plants with and they would live?
Do you inhale while you clean?
Do you use a microwave oven?
Do you cover your food with plastic?

Do you store your food with plastic?
Do you eat canned foods?
Do you have carpeting in your home?
Do you have a memory foam bed?
Do you use commercial household cleaners?
Do you use aluminum cookware?

If you answered yes to any of these questions, you may want to consider an overhaul in your home!

Please refer to my website www.Anti-AgingBody.com for loads of practical information and tips on making your home a wellness sanctuary.

Are Your Skin and Body Care Products Causing Wrinkles?

What creams, lotions, soaps and shampoos do you use? Are they organic? Can you trust the "organic" label on your skincare products? Can you pronounce all the ingredients? Do you know what all the ingredients are? Did you know that organic skincare is not regulated by FDA?

The FDA only regulates food and drugs. Manufacturers can liberally use ingredient labels such as "natural" or "organic" or "herbal" without repercussions. In other words, these labels are essentially meaningless. When you are looking for an organic skin care product, make sure to look for the USDA seal. Skin care falls under the USDA's purview. But, even it the product has the USDA seal and says organic, it is not necessarily safe; make sure to read the list of ingredients.

The skin is our largest organ. It is both an organ of elimination (through sweat) and an organ of absorption. Many people do not realize that the creams, lotions, soaps and shampoos they put on their body are directly absorbed into the blood stream and most of the commercial products on the market are extremely toxic. Nail polishes contain formaldehyde. Formaldehyde is a chemical used in the embalming process! Soaps, shampoos and even toothpaste contain sodium laurel sulfate, a foaming agent. Nearly any product you have that foams up is going to contain this dangerous chemical. Please, read your labels!

Sodium laurel sulfate is a surfactant. The scary thing is that it is used as an engine degreaser. If it cuts through the oil and grime in an engine, imagine its ability to cut through the oils on your scalp and your skin. It gives your hair and skin that squeaky clean feeling; however, it's also stripping the skin of its protective barrier and denaturing the proteins, causing your hair and your skin to be dried out.

If that wasn't bad enough, once it is absorbed into the skin it can mimic an estrogen hormone causing a whole host of new problems. Even worse, this is a substance that cannot even be metabolized by the liver.

Please refer to my website www.Anti-AgingBody.com for an entire series of materials that addresses uncovering hidden toxins in body care products, toxins in your home, pantry and under your sink along with resources for safe alternatives.

Lessons Learned

- Toxins come from many sources including the foods we eat, body care products we use, and as a byproduct of our thoughts and emotions.
- Inflammation and Oxidation are a necessary for a healthy body. It is chronic inflammation and chronic oxidation that are damaging to you. They are a result of cellular stress, most commonly from lack of proper nutrition and stress.

Action Steps

- Implement a diet with more enzyme rich foods such as fresh fruits and vegetables.
- Check out www.Anti-AgingBody.com to learn more about my cleansing programs and alternatives to various cleaning products.

Exercise

I hope this Chapter has caused you to think about the toxins you are exposed to in your daily life, whether they come from food, drink, emotions or your environment. Pick one thing a week to work on, so it becomes a part of your daily routine. For example, Week 1, you may want to take an inventory of what the sources of oxidation and inflammation are in your life. Week 2 you may want to switch out that body moisturizer for a truly nourishing moisturizer, etc.

CHAPTER FIVE

Anti-Aging Food as Medicine

"No illness which can be treated by diet should be treated in any other manner."

Maimonides

"When diet is wrong, medicine is of no use. When diet is correct, medicine is of no need."

Ancient Ayurvedic Proverb

Fake "Food" - The Pathway to Premature Aging and Death

My personal experience, experience with clients and research of scientific studies have taught me that food can be used as a medicine, which has healing properties. Or, food can be a drug, which will cause adverse side effects. Fresh, pure foods, spices and herbs have medicinal properties that nourish and support our body's innate ability to heal. Fake foods act more like a drug in that they cause unwanted symptoms and side effects, causing our bodies to breakdown and become susceptible to illness, disease and premature aging.

As a matter of fact, it is food, stress, environment and emotion that modulate our gene expression. What this means is that our genetics do not dictate or control what disease we may acquire; lifestyle and environmental factors, including our food choices are the determining factors. This is the science of epi- (above) genetics. The science of epigenetics establishes that your genes are not your destiny. You may have a predisposition to something. But, that predisposition does not dictate or guarantee you will acquire that condition. Therefore, it is imperative that we pay attention to our diet and our environment.

Every bite you take will either create an inflammatory response or anti-inflammatory response in your body. There is no doubt that fake "foods" lead to systemic inflammation. Fake foods are processed foods. They are foods filled with preservatives, dyes, artificial colors and flavors. They are made with bleached flour, processed sugar and vegetable oils.

If your diet consists of mostly fake foods, "foods" with no nutritional value like cookies, pastas, doughnuts, breakfast cereals and other processed foods, your body will suffer. Your body will be starving for nutrients, but be overloaded on calories. This is the perfect recipe for weight gain and dis-ease. And, no, "fortified" does not make that "food" nutritious!

These "foods" are just like drugs in that they cause side effects. Our bodies don't know what to do with them. These "foods" cause inflammation, leading us to develop blood sugar spikes, high triglycerides, diabetes, heart disease and certain cancers. They also cause mood disorders, leaky gut syndrome and autoimmune diseases. Every aspect of our body, soul and spirit is affected. The irony is that their side effects cause us to run to the doctor to get a prescription to combat these ills that were self-induced in the first place! Could it be that the food industry is in bed with the pharmaceutical industry?

We have become accustomed to eating fake "foods" on a daily basis. They have become part of the fabric of our society, becoming the norm. We love to bond with family and friends over meals. We "break bread" together. We go out for pizza and beer. We celebrate a birthday with cake, ice-cream and soda. We indulge in "comfort" foods when we are feeling down. We are busy so we go through the drive-thru and eat the burger and fries in our cars, as we are rushing off to the next appointment. After a long day's work we are tired, the kids are hungry and need to buckle down and do their homework. I know; I've been there; it just seems easier to go through the nearest drive-through.

We package and label these items as foods; we refer to them as foods and consume them on a daily basis, but the question no one seems to be asking is: Are these products actually food?

Food is defined as any nourishing substance that is eaten, drunk, or otherwise taken into the body to sustain life, provide energy, promote growth, etc. In my opinion, these items do not meet the definition of food. They do not nourish since they have little to no nutritional value. They fulfill the need to quiet the hunger pangs, but they do not have medicinal value. The truth is that there are a lot of fake foods out there that are quite scary.

Genetically Modified Organisms Cause Age Accelerating Inflammation

One of the scariest fake foods is GMOs. Foods that contain genetically modified ingredients are extremely dangerous for us. Some of the most common genetically modified foods are corn, soy, cotton, canola, yellow crookneck squash, zucchini, papaya and sugar beets. Unless it is organic, you cannot be assured that the food is not genetically modified. When you go to a restaurant, it is extremely likely that you will be consuming a plate full of GMOs, whether they come from the corn on your plate, the oil used to cook your meal or the sugar in your dessert.

There are so many hidden sources of GMOs that it is nearly impossible to avoid them if you are eating packaged foods. Items that contain high fructose corn syrup (HFCS), corn starch, soybean oil, cottonseed oil, and canola oil will all be genetically modified, unless it is clearly labeled as Non-GMO. You will find GMO ingredients in desserts, candies, sautéd vegetables, soy sauce and even vitamin supplements. The list is nearly endless. And, did I mention, there are absolutely no labeling requirements?

But, what is all the fuss? Does it really matter if you eat foods made with GMO vegetable oil? Yes! It is a big deal - even in small amounts. First of all, I don't want someone in a laboratory playing God with my food. Second, it is extremely dangerous to eat these "foods." There is absolutely no testing done to determine the safety of GMOs. Third, it is just plain gross what is being done with our food.

DNA is extracted from bacteria, viruses, insects, fungi, animals or humans and artificially forced into the genes of an unrelated plant or animal. In the case of corn, Monsanto has taken a gene from soil bacteria called Bt (Bacillus thuringiensis), which is a pesticide and spliced it into the DNA of corn, genetically modifying the corn so that the crop will be immune certain insects. The Bt toxin, which is a neurotoxin, is designed to break open the stomach of particular insects, killing them when they bite into the plant. Each plant cell becomes its own toxic pesticide factory which is 1000's times more toxic than if the plant was sprayed with the pesticide. And, to make matters worse, the toxin does not wash off. When you bite into the corn or corn product, the Bt toxin goes to work on you and shreds your digestive tract. It doesn't distinguish between a bug, a small child or an adult. A neurotoxin is a neurotoxin. It is designed to kill, and it does its job. It may just take a bit longer to kill a human.

There is a false sense of safety with these crops. Many people don't realize the FDA does not test GMOs for their safety. In the United States, our government has taken the position that it will allow GMOs into our food supply since they have not been proven to be unsafe. Contrast this with Europe, which has taken the approach that unless they are proven to be safe, they will not allow GMOs into their food supply. Our government's position has forever tainted the landscape of our farmlands. GMOs have cross-contaminated and tainted non-GMO crops.

As I mentioned, the FDA does not conduct studies to ensure that GMOs are safe. However, a study in Quebec has concluded that the Bt toxin was found in the blood of 93% of pregnant women and 80% of umbilical blood of their babies! The ramifications of this are staggering. Since the blood-brain barrier is not developed in fetuses and newborns, the toxin can cause or contribute to severe cognitive problems, such as autism. If the toxin attacks the gut lining, autoimmune disease could result.

The American Medical Association's policy is one that "supports the FDA's science-based approach to special product labeling, recognizing that there currently is no evidence that there are material differences or safety concerns in available bioengineered foods. Recognizing the public's interest in the safety of bioengineered foods, the new policy also supports mandatory FDA pre-market systemic safety assessments of these foods as a preventive measure to ensure the health of the public. We also urge the FDA to remain alert to new data on the health consequences of bioengineered foods."

This sounds great, right? The AMA supports the "FDA's science-based approach." It sounds like the AMA is aware of the FDA conducting their own studies on GMOs - and those studies prove GMOs are safe, doesn't it? In my opinion, the AMA is grossly abdicating their responsibility and failing in their stated mission to "promote the art and science of medicine and the betterment of public health," especially since the FDA has not and is not conducting any of their own "science-based" safety tests of their own on GMOs.

This lack of testing is due to a decades old policy that gives authority the biotech companies to determine the safety of their GMO foods. The FDA issued a meaningless statement that read "we recognize and appreciate the strong interest that many consumers have in knowing whether a food was produced using genetic engineering. The FDA supports voluntary labeling for food derived from genetic engineering. Currently, food manufacturers may indicate through voluntary labeling whether foods have or have not been developed through genetic engineering provided that such labeling is truthful and not misleading."

Again, other countries hold to the policy that GMOs must be proven safe before they are introduced into the market; while the US holds to the policy that GMOs are safe until proven otherwise. Clearly, the FDA's allegiance is to the biotech companies, not to its stated mission of "protecting and promoting your health." It is the biotech companies that are making billions in profits from GMOs in conduct their own "voluntary safety consultations."

Because I do not trust the government authorities to protect my health and welfare, I advise my clients buy only organic products or products labeled "Non-GMO." I also instruct my clients to read all food labels. If a label list ingredients that contain the words corn, soy, canola or cottonseed oil, put it back on the shelf. If it is made with beet sugar, don't buy it. Over 80% of non-organic processed, grocery store foods contain GMOs. These "foods" are dangerous, they are toxic, and they expose you and your family to developing devastating diseases, which results in unnecessary heartache and pain. They should not be consumed at all. It is time we vote with our dollars and refuse GMOs.

Additives and Preservatives - They Preserve the Food, Not You

Additives and preservatives are great - for the food manufacturer, that is. They want their product to have a long shelf life. Clearly, they are not concerned with your shelf life. The bottom line is that additives and preservatives are not fit for human consumption.

Let's take a look at fake foods that contain fake or altered fat. Food manufacturers have manipulated Omega 6 rich oils from corn, cottonseed, safflower, sunflower and soy to create unhealthy convenience foods.

The Omega 6 overload leads to brain inflammation, bad moods and blood clots. An inflamed brain does not lead to a youthful, nimble body or brain. In fact, its just the opposite. An inflamed brain certainly leads to accelerated aging, Alzheimer's disease and dementia.

Not only that, the Omega 6 overload contributes to the aging of our skin, causing wrinkles and loss of elasticity, and aging of our internal organs. For years margarine and trans-fats had been promoted as "heart healthy" fats. After decades of being fed this lie by food manufacturers, their experimentation with the US population, and after countless preventable heart attacks and deaths, in November 2013 our government has finally declared that these products are no longer "generally regarded as safe" and proposed a ban on them.

The FDA's deputy commissioner for foods said that there is not a timetable for the ban, but "we want to do it in a way that doesn't unduly disrupt markets." We have a "proposed" ban without a timeline on a substance that is known to cause disease and early death. Additionally, we have loopholes created by the FDA allowing food manufacturers to continue to include trans fats in their packaged food, labeling them "trans fat free" if the serving size has less than 0.5 grams per serving. How many consumers check the food label and only eat one serving of that packaged food?

Call me naive, but isn't the FDA supposed to protect our health rather than the food manufacturer's bottom line? This is an outrage! Our government is finally letting us know that these products are no longer regarded as safe. On their own website, they acknowledge that "reducing trans fat intake could prevent thousands of heart attacks and deaths." Why aren't trans fats pulled off the market now? Today? Whose interests are they protecting?

Read your food labels. Look for the word "hydrogenated." This is a clue that the product contains trans fats. If you see "hydrogenated" on the label, but the item back on the shelf.

Meat Glue

Considering the government's stance on trans-fats, it comes as no surprise that the FDA and USDA have readily approved of the use of transglutaminase, which is commonly referred to as meat glue. Meat glue is an enzyme that is derived from fermented bacteria or animal blood. Meat glue has been used in commercial processing to bind proteins together. It is used in making imitation crab meat, fish balls, processed meat and binding together meat scraps. Just because you don't eat meat doesn't mean you are safe from meat glue. It is also used to thicken egg yolks, strengthen dough, improve tofu texture and make milk and yogurt products creamier. The fact that most transglutaminase is made with animal blood means that it is not kosher.

Lots of chefs use it. How do you think that bacon strip stays glued to that tasty filet mignon? Yep, it's the meat glue! It can also be used to strengthen noodles that are low in gluten, such as buckwheat soba noodles. Most commonly it is used in bonding nice scraps of meat together. The danger of this is that bacteria can get trapped between the pieces of meat. If you enjoy a rare steak, you could be exposing yourself to food poisoning.

Chefs are getting creative in using it to make their culinary creations. Due to modern technology and the advancement of transglutaminase it is getting more and more difficult to detect if the product has been processed with meat glue.

When the meat is cooked, there is no way to tell if your food has been prepared with this. This is just one more reason to only eat organic food products. It is my opinion that any time food is processed or modified, we end up paying the consequences with our physical, mental and emotional health.

Egg Beaters

It is interesting to see how food manufacturers manipulate foods under the auspices of making them healthier for us, as if our creator didn't know what he was doing in the first place. Whenever the scientist in the lab invents a new "health" food, time has shown that he should have just stayed out of the kitchen in the first place. It is ironic that the designer "health" food usually turns out to cause inflammation, heart disease or cancer. Some classic examples are saccharine, olestra, trans-fats and aspartame.

How many times have you looked over a menu and noticed "heart healthy" choices? One item on that menu will be an omelet made with Egg Beaters. Dr. Fred Kummerow, of the University of Illinois, published a study in Pediatrics 1974, entitled Nutritional Value of Egg Beaters Compared With "Farm Fresh Eggs." Despite Egg Beaters being heavily promoted as a heart healthy food, the evidence was overwhelming that Egg Beaters were anything but heart healthy.

Rats were divided into two groups. One group was fed exclusively fresh eggs, including the yolk, while the other group of rats was fed exclusively Egg Beaters. The rats fed the whole egg were healthy, grew normally and were able to reproduce. The rats that were fed Egg Beaters only were malnourished, did not grow to full size, were in ill health, not able to reproduce, and all died before reaching maturity. This study clearly demonstrated just how deleterious fake foods are to our health.

Waxed Fruits and Vegetables - No, Not the Ones Used for Household Decorations

All of us love beautiful things. We want beautiful homes, cars and bodies. We also want beautiful looking fruits and vegetables. One way to get that beautiful crisp salad or shiny red, ripe tomato is to use wax. Can we trust the FDA to step in and protect us?

According to the FDA website, coatings used on fruits and vegetables must meet the FDA additive regulations for safety. There are certain approved coatings for vegetables, including petroleum, beeswax, or shellac from the Lac beetle, modified atmospheric packaging (MAP), edible biodegradable coatings, and plasticizers to maintain freshness. Doesn't that all sound yummy?

Most of the time consumers don't even know the wax is on the produce. All we know is that we want the freshest ingredients possible. We instinctively reach for the most vibrant, brightest, unblemished pieces of produce and crisp leafy greens. It seems logical to assume that if you chooses the prettiest piece of produce that it is the healthiest piece as well. However, it may be that the color and freshness are sealed in with wax.

You may be thinking that you are not impacted by the waxy coating because you wash your salad fixings. Surely you are safe. However, the only way to completely remove the wax from the fruit or vegetable is to peel the skin. There are some lettuces that have been treated with this wax and you can actually peel off the wax. How do you think that "fresh" McDonald's salad stays looking so beautiful and crisp all day long?

In addition to just not wanting to eat the shellac, the danger with the wax is bacteria can get caught underneath it. This means that even though you wash your produce, you may be unknowingly eating your lettuce with bacteria. Many of the waxes are petroleum based and inorganic. Your body does not know what to do with petroleum or petroleum based products.

You can find more information with regard to food labeling and my buyer's guide on my website, www.Anti-AgingBody.com.

Gluten

Gluten is found in wheat, barley, rye and a few other grains. It is also found in unlikely products such as beer, licorice, imitation seafood, gravy, sauces, soy sauce and marinades.

Gluten is a vegetable protein that gives elasticity and a chewy texture to dough. It is also called seitan, which is commonly used as a meat substitute due to its texture. Even though our government recommends we consume a diet rich in grains, I think we have learned by now that the FDA doesn't have our best interest at heart when it comes to what we put in our mouths. We will be well served to completely avoid all forms of gluten. Whole wheat bread is not a health food by any stretch of the imagination. Whether or not you have Celiac's Disease, gluten is something that our bodies cannot digest.

Celiac's disease is an autoimmune disease that is triggered by the consumption of gluten. Many people also have a condition called Non-Celiac Gluten Sensitivity (NCGS). This condition can be even more dangerous than Celiac's disease because as it goes undiagnosed the gut, organs and even the brain continue to be damaged due to the continued consumption of gluten.

The ramifications of having this condition and not realizing the long-term damaging effects of gluten, can slowly erode and devastate our health. Our bodies cannot digest the gluten. Over time gut permeability or leaky gut develops. Gut permeability means that large proteins are able to pass through the small intestines directly into the bloodstream.

The gut permeability leads to inflammation in the gut, creating symptoms that aren't necessarily associated with digestive issues. It is insidious. Inflammation can be raging inside of us, leading to a whole host of autoimmune diseases like rheumatoid arthritis or Hashimoto's disease.

Gluten consumption can trigger a myriad of symptoms such as brain fog, irritability and even neurological problems.

My client Suzanne had a long history of weight issues, depression, intermittent diarrhea and brain fog. She had no enthusiasm for life.

She seemed to be doing everything right, changing her diet, exercising and she even began meditating. Her symptoms persisted. We uncovered that she was consuming hidden sources of gluten. Once she completely eliminated gluten from her diet, her digestion stabilized and her mood lifted. The gluten, even in minute amounts affected every aspect of her life. She now has her life back!

Research has shown that if you have NCGS, that inflammation can occur in your brain. This inflammation can result in lesions on the brain which will impede your path to health, happiness and enlightenment.

Foods for a Youthful, Sexy Body

That's it for the bad news. I hope I have made my case against fake foods. It is easy to see that man-made, fake foods will lead you to a broken down and possibly diseased body and mind. Clearly, a diet high in these foods will not help you turn back the hands of time. Most certainly, they will lead to chronic inflammation which will accelerate the aging process.

The good news is that there are foods that do heal your body, mind and spirit, halting and reversing the aging process. These are fresh, pure foods; foods that are living and have enzyme activity; foods that have not been heated to over 105 to 118 degrees Fahrenheit. They are organic, and they have high vibrational energy. I look at foods from a little different perspective from most diet or nutrition books on the market. I look at the food from the perspective of their vibrational energy.

As Einstein said, "Everything is energy . . . Match the frequency of the reality you want and you cannot help but get that reality . . . This is not philosophy. This is physics."

The highest vibrational foods are foods that are naturally nutrient dense and rich in color. Marine phytoplankton is one of the Earth's most nutrient dense alkaline foods on the planet. This food has directly absorbed the energy from the sun and transmuted that energy into its DNA. The same is true with spirulina, plus this has an extremely high concentration of bio-available protein.

Other high vibration foods include dark, green leafy vegetables because they contain chlorophyll which is synthesized sunlight. This is exceptionally purifying for our blood. And our blood is the life-force of our body. Chlorophyll is one of the supplements I used to reverse my Crohn's disease.

Goji berries are another high vibrational food. They help support the immune system, have anti-aging properties, support eye health, energy levels and enhance your mood. All of these benefits tie right into our quest for youthfulness.

Another extremely high vibrational food is raw cacao. I want to emphasize that it must be raw since once it is processed it becomes a different substance. When it is in its raw state, cacao has an extremely high vibration. It is high in anti-oxidants, in fact one of the top antioxidant foods on the planet. It has over 300 identifiable chemical compounds making it one of the most nutritionally complex foods on earth. Cacao helps support our heart and cardiovascular health. The health benefits don't stop there. Raw cacao affects our emotional state by lifting our mood.

When making food choices, it is important to look at how we want to feel and determine what we want to accomplish. In other words, what is your target? Compare this to where you are in this moment. Now figure out how to get from point A to point B. Let's reverse engineer our diets: consider the compounds that will lift our moods, raise our vibrational energy, extinguish the inflammation and reverse the aging process. Let's incorporate these foods in our diets on a daily basis. By doing this on a regular basis, you will inevitably increase your vitality and raise your vibrational energy.

The foods and beverages that you consume are the building blocks of your body. What you eat and drink becomes your brain, your blood, muscles and organs. If you do not have the health or the body that you want, take a hard look at what is on your plate.

Lessons Learned

- Just because a certain product is labeled as healthy, it does not mean that it is. Read the ingredients on the label, checking for additives and preservatives.
- GMOs are the most dangerous fake food on the market. They are not labeled, so purchase food products that are labeled "organic" or "Non-GMO Verified."

Action Steps

- Look at the ingredients contained in the foods you eat, including the meals you order at a restaurant.
- Eliminate gluten from your diet.

Exercise

I hope this Chapter has caused you to think about the food your have in your pantry and refrigerator. Pick one thing a week to work on, so it becomes a part of your daily routine. For example, Week 1, you may want to read the labels on each food item you consume, making note of the products that contain ingredients you are unfamiliar with. Week 2 you may want to switch out vegetable oil with organic coconut oil, etc.

CHAPTER SIX

Anti-Aging Basics For Every Diet

"If there is magic on this planet, it is contained in water."

Loran Eisley

No matter what philosophy you subscribe to, no matter what diet you follow, there are certain basics that apply across the board. Each person needs the same basic macronutrients: fats, proteins and carbohydrates. We need good quality fats for a healthy brain and cell membrane integrity. We need proteins for building muscle and manufacturing neurotransmitters. We need carbohydrates to supply energy to each of our cells. We need fiber to ensure everything moves through our bodies and we can eliminate toxins. And, we need to stay hydrated given that we are approximately 70% water.

It is important to remember that brain health and youthfulness go hand in hand. If the brain tissue is compromised, halting the aging process will be elusive. So, lets delve right in.

Water

Water is basic to our existence. Approximately 3/4 of the earth is made up of water. Plant, animal and human life are all dependent upon it. We cannot survive for more than a week without water. Water is essential to flushing out toxins from our bodies. It helps us assimilate nutrients, carries oxygen to each and every cell.

Dehydration causes fatigue, fuzzy memory, difficulty focusing and lightheadedness. It is ironic that when suffering from these symptoms, the masses turn to the very things that cause further exacerbate the problem. They turn to coffee, soda or energy drinks to perk them up. These may give us a jolt but end up dehydrating us, exacerbating the problem. Also, dehydration can mimic hunger. So, when you feel hunger, try drinking a glass of fresh spring water and see if the hunger pangs go away.

There are volumes that discuss the importance of clean, pure water. I want to touch on another aspect of water that is just as powerful in promoting health. Masaru Emoto, the author of, "The Hidden Messages in Water", demonstrated that water molecules actually changed their very structure after being exposed to thoughts. It did not matter if those thoughts were positive or negative; the structure of the water was changed. He demonstrated that water actually absorbs the energy of the thoughts you think.

In the study, when people expressed their thoughts of gratitude, the water crystals took on beautiful, symmetrical shapes. When people expressed thoughts of hate or anger, the water crystals took on asymmetrical, misshapen and chaotic structures. Given this, I believe it is important to prepare your foods with love and gratitude.

It is amazing to realize that the structure of your water can change with the power of your thoughts of gratitude. It just makes sense to express gratitude for what you eat and drink prior to consuming it, especially when eating foods that are high in water content.

Most religions and spiritual practices teach giving thanks for the food before you eat. People talk about preparing meals with love. There is something basic and at the same time profound in incorporating this practice in our daily lives.

The quality of your water matters. When you drink water and its subtle energies, it will be transmuted into your blood. The best water to drink is fresh, spring water that has not been touched by human hands. Water that is pure, has not been tainted with fluoride or chlorine. The water that I personally drink, I found after doing research and looking at the website, www.findaspring.com. I will go to the spring with my five gallon glass jugs, fill them, and bring them home. I drink and cook with this water.

Fats Keep Your Skin and Mind Young

Fats are a critical component to our health, well-being and youthfulness. Fats are the building blocks of the membranes of each and every cell of our body. Our brains are about 2/3 fat. Your brain weighs approximately 3 pounds or about 2% of your total body weight. It has 100 billion neurons and over 100,000 miles of blood vessels. It uses 20% of the oxygen and 20% of the glucose you consume. The brain down through the spinal cord is encased in a protective coating called the myelin sheath. The myelin sheath is 70% fat and 30% protein. Considering your brain and central nervous system controls just about every bodily function, along with your decisions and daily choices, feelings and emotions, having the best quality building blocks is non-negotiable.

The question becomes, what are you using to build your cells? What are you using to form your brain? Not all fats are created equal.

There are good fats and bad fats. Good fats lead to health and wellness, while bad fats lead to degeneration, sickness, accelerated aging and disease. So, what are the good fats? It is pretty safe to ignore what the TV commercials tell us. Trans-fats and margarine were heavily promoted as great for your heart and for weight loss. We now know that they are deadly. Saturated fats have been vilified. However, we have scientific evidence that proves otherwise. The evidence proves that the right saturated fats lead to health and wellness.

A basic philosophy of mine is that every time man touches a food to "improve" upon it, we manage to mess it up. It will be promoted as a health food, then inevitably the evidence will come out that the product is toxic. Take saccharine, GMOs or chlorinated, fluoridated water for example. Now, trans-fats. Lets just stop trying to improve upon what God has already created.

Lets go a little deeper into reasons why fats are so important and critical to our health. Every single cell membrane, is made up of essential fatty acids along with proteins. The function of the cell membrane is to allow oxygen, glucose, and micronutrients in. At the same time, the membrane is semi-permeable and allows the metabolic waste to exit thus keeping the cell from polluting itself. If lipid component of the cell wall is made up of processed fats, the membrane becomes rigid and inflexible. It no longer has the same degree of permeability.

Bad fats are trans fats, hydrogenated oils, or PUFA (poly unsaturated fatty acids). A diet rich in these manipulated fats and oils means that you will be forced to use these substandard materials to build your cell membranes and brain tissue. When forced to use the trans fats and PUFAs to build our cell membranes, the membrane becomes brittle and impermeable. Cells don't absorb the nutrients they need for survival. Receptor sites on the cell membrane don't function properly either.

For example, cells have receptor sites for insulin. This is what drives the glucose in the bloodstream into the cell. If the receptor site is compromised, the insulin can't drive the glucose into the cell. The cell will begin to starve. Symptoms of diabetes will develop. In addition to the cells not getting the nutrition they need, they can't eliminate the metabolic waste from within. Then premature cell death occurs due to autointoxication or pollution. Your cells become toxic and you accelerate the aging process. Your skin loses elasticity and easily wrinkles. You look old.

When you think about it, if a trans fatty acid is incorporated into the cell membrane, the cell membrane becomes rigid and is no longer semi permeable causing oxidative damage. Completely eliminating all bad fats and incorporating only good fats into our diets is essential to young, healthy skin and reversing the inflammation that leads to accelerated aging.

When trying to decipher between good fats and bad fats, consider whether it has been processed, cooked or heated. One of the main concerns with fats and oils is that when cooked or heated, the molecular structure changes and they become foreign to your body. If it is foreign to your body, and your body doesn't know what to do with it, it is toxic.

Scientific data is conclusive, trans-fatty acids are extremely toxic on many levels. They negatively impact the brain by affecting the brain's electrical activity, disrupting the communication on a cellular level. Trans-fats cause cellular degeneration, resulting in diminished mental performance, premature sagging and wrinkling of the skin.

It is best to eat foods as close to their natural state as possible, especially fats. When extracting the oil from the nut or seed, heat is involved. Oils quickly become rancid. If you are going to consume oils, even olive oil, you need to get cold pressed virgin or extra virgin olive oil. One of the things to be aware of, especially with regard to olive oil, is that the industry is not regulated. Often times you might think you are buying a quality olive oil based upon the label saying it is "pure" or "natural" and it is not. They may have cut it with other oils that are not healthful at all.

I purchased "pure olive oil" that was "carefully pressed from olives" and discovered that it was anything but pure and not fit for human consumption. One simple test to determine whether or not you actually have olive oil is to pour a bit of the oil into a dish or glass and put it into the refrigerator. If it solidifies, you may not know the quality, but at least you know it is olive oil. Other oils such as canola oil or vegetable oils do not solidify when you refrigerate them. So many commercial brand olive oils are cut with cheaper oils for greater profit margins, and the label does not disclose that information. You just cannot trust the packaging when it comes to olive oil. You must do some research and contact the manufacturer. You can refer to my website www.Anti-AgingBody.com for further information and resources.

The good fats are the essential fatty acids; the Omega 3s and Omega 6s. Where do we get these essential fatty acids from? And, are we eating them in the correct ratio?

Some of the healthy good fats that need to be incorporated into our diets come from avocado, olives and coconut. Coconut oil is one of the most versatile, healthful fats available. Sources of Omega 3s include chia seeds, walnuts, leafy greens and sea vegetables. The healthy Omega 6s come from sesame oil. The brain uses these raw ingredients to make DHA and arachidonic acid.

It is clear when looking at what the brain needs for optimal health that diet is essential. Diet directly affects the brain. It affects the chemicals and influences mood, behavior, thought and emotions. An unhealthy brain has low DHA levels. This results in neurodegeneration. What this means to you, is that fatty acid loss can contribute to Alzheimer's disease and Parkinson's disease. Low DHA levels have been associated with hostility and aggression.

But it isn't only "bad" fats that compromise the health of your tissues. Stress, alcohol, sugar, vitamin or mineral deficiencies all lead to the degradation of your health on a cellular level. What results then is oxidative damage, cognitive impairment ultimately leading to depression.

Psychology Today published an article which detailed a study that consisted of one million students. A portion of the students were restricted from artificial flavors, dyes or preservatives in their school lunches These students did 14% better on IQ tests than those who ate lunches laced with artificial flavors, dyes and preservatives. This study clearly demonstrated the power of a proper diet and its impact on your brain and intelligence.

Protein for a Sharp Mind

When we are talking about maintaining a youthful, sharp brain, we need to think about the brain and how it functions. We have incorporated the healthy fats in our diets so that we can develop healthy brain tissue; we must also address our neurotransmitters. They are the chemical substances that transmit information from neuron to neuron and other cells in the body. Basically, the neurotransmitters allow the brain cells to communicate information throughout the body and within the brain.

One class of neurotransmitters is made from amino acids. Amino acids are the building blocks of protein. There are several types of neurotransmitters. In fact, to date, there are more than 100 chemical messengers that have been identified. Each is interdependent upon the other. The key to strive for is balance.

The balance is so intricate, that manipulating this balance through drugs can become a prescription for disaster. Since food affect us just like a drug, it is advised to turn to diet first, before running to the doctor for that prescription.

The functions of neurotransmitters are extensive. They tell our heart to beat, our lungs to breathe, regulate our mood, our sleep, and modulate our weight levels. They are affected by stress, diet, neurotoxins, drugs, alcohol, caffeine and environmental toxins.

Our brains are very sensitive, electrically charged organs. They are responsible for growth, development, moods and enlightenment. That is why it is important that we give our brain everything that it needs so it can function optimally. Just living in our society, we are exposing our brains and central nervous system to a daily electrical assault from electro-magnetic radiation, Wi-Fi and smart meters. These energies do interfere with the electrical current of the brain.

It is indisputable that our brains are very susceptible to dietary and environmental exposures around us. Likewise, healthy, balanced neurotransmitters are susceptible as well. Since we are bombarded with environmental stimuli that interferes with our brain's electrical circuitry, it is of utmost importance to focus on things in our control, like nutrition. Our diets influence healthy, balanced neurotransmitters.

There are two categories of neurotransmitters I would like to focus on: Those that are inhibitory which calm you and those that are excitatory which stimulate you. Some of the key neurotransmitters in these categories are dopamine, serotonin and GABA. Dopamine modulates mood, GABA regulates anxiety and serotonin plays a role in depression, suicide, aggression and impulsive behavior.

One amino acid, tyrosine, will increase the production of dopamine, epinephrine and norepinephrine, increasing energy and alertness. Tryptophan is a precursor of serotonin. It is interesting to note that low carbohydrate diets tend to lead to depression. Insulin is released in the blood stream after eating carbohydrates. This clears the blood of most amino acids, except for tryptophan. The tryptophan then crosses the blood brain barrier, ultimately depleting the tryptophan in the blood, leading to decreased serotonin, and depression. As you can see, the balance is extremely complex. Regulating our neurotransmitters via prescription medication is next to impossible and will with throw the delicate balance off.

When considering neurotransmitter balance, some of the top offenders are coffee and alcohol. Coffee is detrimental to the delicate balance because it depletes epinephrine. However, when you consume your cup of coffee, it will give you that little caffeine high giving you a false sense of energy and boost in your mood.

Alcohol is detrimental to the delicate balance because it depletes GABA production. The effects of alcohol are deceptive. When you first drink the alcohol, it has a tendency to relax you, creating an initial feeling of relaxation. GABA depletion leads to higher anxiety levels.

To help with serotonin levels, I recommend a diet rich in avocado, banana, red plums, tomatoes, pineapple, eggplant, and walnuts.

I also suggest a diet rich in nutrients that support the body in making neurotransmitters, such as folic acid found in leafy greens and citrus foods; B-6 found in bell peppers, squash and turnip greens; biotin found in Swiss chard, walnuts and berries; bio-available iron found in dark, leafy greens and dried fruit; and pantothenic acid (B-5) found in sunflower seeds, avocado, and mushrooms.

Again, don't ignore lifestyle choices. Stop smoking, cut out sugar and caffeine, white flour, and junk foods. I recommend working on stabilizing your blood sugar levels by incorporating exercise and stress management techniques. I also assist my clients in detecting food allergies or sensitivities and correcting any nutritional deficiencies.

I have found that when clients get the right nutrition, are able to assimilate their nutrients, and have proper elimination, everything in their life improves. They make better choices, enjoy mental clarity and lead happier lives.

Carbohydrates Keep You Going Strong

Carbohydrates fall into two basic categories: simple carbohydrates and complex carbohydrates. The simple carbohydrates breakdown quickly into glucose causing spikes in your blood glucose level - resulting in insulin spikes. Examples include grains, pastas, processed foods and breads. These are the carbohydrates to work towards eliminating from your diet. It is the complex carbohydrates that are healthful to your body as they supply a steady source of glucose, without causing spikes in your blood sugar levels. These are the carbohydrates which are contained in vegetables and whole fruits. They are essential for health and longevity as they break down slowly, releasing a steady stream of glucose into the bloodstream. They are essential to your body and mind as are nourishing and health producing.

Carbohydrates are an important component for our diet and for our brain. However, our brain does not use carbohydrates as a building block like it uses fats. Carbohydrates cannot be made into neurotransmitters, either. They do, however supply the glucose that is necessary for the brain to operate. Glucose is the fuel that is used by the brain. Considering the brain cannot store glucose, it is reliant on a steady fuel supply via the bloodstream.

The brain is a glucose hog. It needs two times the energy as other cells. Even though it is a glucose hog, sugars and refined carbs actually deplete the energy supply. Diets high in sugar or refined carbs cause blood sugar spikes, resulting in insulin being released to lower the blood sugar levels. Thus creating a scarcity of glucose in the bloodstream.

Sugar spikes wreak havoc on your entire body. With too little glucose, your body doesn't have adequate energy to synthesize key neurotransmitters. With too much glucose in the bloodstream, it taxes the liver. There is a cascade effect. Insulin is released, and glucose level is normalized. You may think all is good because the glucose level has gone down, but its not. Insulin levels are still high in the bloodstream, the liver cannot metabolize the insulin fast enough, creating insulin resistance which is then tied to neurodegeneration.

It is also a rather new discovery that the brain itself produces insulin. The drop in insulin production in the brain contributes to degeneration of brain cells which can lead to conditions such as Alzheimer's disease and plaque in the brain. In fact, some experts refer to Alzheimer's disease as Type 3 Diabetes. In order to reduce insulin resistance and susceptibility to conditions such as Alzheimer's, it is important to avoid high glycemic substances such as sugar, grain and fructose. I also recommend avoiding agave syrup.

Fiber - The Unsung Hero in Anti-Aging Strategies

There are two types of dietary fiber: soluble and insoluble. Both are indispensable to your health and wellbeing. They have different functions. Fiber is essential to your health because it can lower cholesterol, help with weight loss, prevent constipation and colon cancer, and improve digestion. In a Harvard study of over 40,000 male health professionals, researchers found that a high total dietary fiber intake was linked to a 40% lower risk of coronary heart disease, compared to a low-fiber intake.

Let's talk about insoluble fiber first. This is known as roughage, or the indigestible portion of the fruit or vegetable. It is best to eat whole fruits, rather than juice them because the fiber slows down the digestion process and decreases blood sugar spikes from the fructose in the fruit. A diet rich in fruit juices, even if they are freshly squeezed, will cause blood sugar spikes. And as we have already discussed, the blood sugar spikes over time can and will have adverse effects on your health.

Insoluble fiber helps to keep the food moving though the digestive tract. The result will be regular, soft bowel movements. If someone is constipated, the waste from digested food remains in the colon too long. The body will absorb the toxins from the waste and cause autointoxication. This puts a great burden on the liver and all the other organs. People can become very ill from the autointoxication.

Studies have shown that soluble fiber reduces the absorption of cholesterol in your intestines by binding with bile and dietary cholesterol so that the body excretes it. Juicing vegetables and going on a vegetable juice fast is a great way to reduce the cholesterol that has built up in your arteries.

Some tips for increasing your daily dietary fiber intake is to eat high fiber foods throughout the day. Eat a piece of fruit as a snack during the day. Eat a mix of vegetables on your salad or cut up some fresh vegetables to snack on throughout the day. Make sure to drink plenty of water through the day as well. This will ensure the fiber keeps moving through your system.

Incorporate foods that do double duty. For example, avocados are a great source of soluble and insoluble fiber, as well as healthy fats. Raspberries are another great source of fiber, as well as antioxidants. For females, aim for 25 grams of fiber a day; if you are male, aim for 35 - 40 grams of fiber per day.

Supplements for Strong, Supple Bodies

I think that the best way to get the nutrients that your body needs is directly through your food. This is because your food is much more than just macronutrients and micronutrients. Pure, whole food has fiber. It also has cofactors which are chemical compounds that are required to activate the bioactivity of the foods you eat. And fruits, vegetables, nuts and seeds all have powerful phytonutrients and enzymes, most of which haven't even been discovered yet.

What we have done is isolate and extract the vitamins and minerals we have identified and put them in a pill. Corporations have made synthetic versions of these substances and marketed them to us in the form of a vitamin supplement, or "fortified" our bread and cereal with them.

However, it is impossible to get the same benefit out of an isolated vitamin as out of a fresh piece of produce since not all the phytonutrients and co-factors will be included in the pill. That said, I also know that our soils are depleted. Our soils are not the same soils that existed 50 years ago. Further, if you buy conventionally grown foods they are going to be grown with petroleum based fertilizers. There is no doubt, these crops will not be of the same high nutrient value when they are being doused with petroleum based fertilizers, when compared to organic produce. Again, just one more reason why it is very important to have your diet consist of organic foods.

Since our soils are depleted and since it is important that we get the proper nutrients, sometimes supplementation is essential. I advise my clients to make sure that their supplements are made from organic ingredients. One of the dirty secrets in the supplement industry is that a lot of supplements are made with GMO ingredients. This is something that is not being regulated as there are no laws mandating the labeling of GMO ingredients on a product.

Another dirty secret is that most commercial brand vitamins are made from coal-tar derivatives. Our bodies are not designed like a car engine. It does not know what to do with petroleum based products.

My rule-of-thumb when I buy supplements is to make sure they are from a professional line and they are organic. A word on the professional lines; professional lines are developed for efficacy.

These companies want to make sure that the product works versus a warehouse store brand product. Most products that are sold at a supermarket or vitamin store are formulated and designed to sell large volume. They use slick advertising to promote the product without regard to you, the consumer.

One example of this marketing is with fish oils. Fish oil supplements are promoted as a healthy way to get your Omega 3's. However, what I have observed as a selling point for some fish oils is that it will not "repeat" on you. Meaning you will not taste it or you will not burp it up after you swallow the capsule. A lot of people see this as a great selling point. I am sure these companies are selling more product, but they are not doing anything to enhance your health. The problem with this fish oil is that the capsule was made so that it would not open until it was pretty far down in the small intestine.

That's an issue because fats and oils get broken down and absorbed higher in your intestinal tract. All oils and fats need to be "emulsified" with bile, which is injected into the digestive tract in the duodenum. The bile acts as a degreaser, allowing the body to breakdown the fats and oils into fatty acids which are essential to health and youthful appearance.

If you took this product, you would not be getting the benefit from the fish oil. Instead you are pooping it out. The best case scenario in taking cheap supplements is that you have expensive poop and pee. The worst case scenario is that these supplements become toxic, causing chronic inflammation and oxidation, leading to accelerated aging of your skin and organs.

For more information regarding supplementation you can go to the resources page on my website at www.Anti-AgingBody.com.

Protecting Your Gut with Probiotics and Prebiotics

Have you ever heard that expression "you have a gut feeling," or "go with your gut," or "what does your gut say," "butterflies in your stomach?" There is a reason for that. Your gut is your second brain. It consists of one hundred million neurons, which is more than what you have in the spinal cord. Up to 95% of the serotonin is produced in the gut not in the brain.

The second brain, your gut, influences mood, emotions, behavior, thoughts, aggression and depression. It is critical that we nourish our gut flora. A healthy gut full of life enhancing bacteria. In fact, your gut has more DNA from bacteria than your own human DNA.

Bacteria are essential to our health and emotional wellbeing because it helps to complete the digestive process. A byproduct of the bacteria is that it produces vitamins.

I recommend addressing gut health from two perspectives. First, stop causing an imbalance with our gut flora due to using antibiotics, chlorinated water, antibacterial soaps, agriculture chemicals, pesticides and herbicides. Second, repopulate and feed the beneficial bacteria.

Diet plays an integral role in the health of our gut flora. Think about it. If you eat conventionally grown foods they have been sprayed with insecticides and herbicides. These chemicals are designed to kill living organisms, bacteria and pathogens. However, these chemicals don't discriminate. They are equal opportunity killers. They will kill the healthy gut flora. Washing your produce is not enough.

These chemicals are especially dangerous when you realize that 80% of your immune system is in your gut. Some of indications of an imbalance of your gut flora are sugar cravings, gas, and digestive issues. If you have a sugar craving that you just cannot get over, chances are extremely high that is not your weak willpower, but it is an imbalance in your gut flora.

It is the dysbiosis, the imbalance of the gut flora, the candida overgrowth that is crying out for sugar. The candida feeds off of sugar. When you have a diet that is high in processed foods, high in starchy foods, high in sugar, the candida is going to flourish.

This imbalance will directly impact the serotonin levels in the gut. It is interesting to note that common side effects of antidepressants which are SSRI's or serotonin reuptake inhibitors is that they provoke side effects in your gastrointestinal tract.

There are so many tools to use to help cultivate healthy gut flora. Eating cultured or fermented foods on a daily basis is great. However, don't rush out just yet and buy your favorite supermarket yogurt. You probably won't be doing your body any favors. Most yogurt manufacturers add a lot of sugar, HFCS or artificial sweeteners, along with stabilizers which end up completely defeating the purpose of eating the yogurt in the first place. You are eating the yogurt to repopulate and feed the good bacteria; the sugar defeats the purpose, feeding the candida, contributing to the dysbiosis.

Sauerkraut and kimchee are really great fermented foods, however if you go to the supermarket chances are they are going to be pasteurized. This means that all the medicinal benefits of these foods are cooked out. The beneficial bacteria are killed in the pasteurization process.

There are solutions to ensuring you are able to correct any gut dysbiosis you may have. The first step is eliminating sugar from your diet. Second, supplementation with professional grade probiotics (see the Resources section on my website www.Anti-AgingBody.com). Third, making your own sauerkraut, kimchee, or yogurt. Or, if you do buy these products, make sure you buy them raw and unpasteurized. FInally, make sure you feed the beneficial gut flora with prebiotics.

Prebiotics are a type of plant fiber that nourishes the beneficial bacteria in the gut. Foods that contain prebiotics include beans, raw garlic, raw onion, Jerusalem artichoke, jicama, dandelion and chicory root.

Enzymes Are the Spark of Life

Another basic for a healthy diet is enzyme supplementation. Again, enzymes are the spark of life. They are necessary to break down the macronutrients so our bodies can access the micronutrients and phytonutrients. They are essential in helping our bodies assimilate and utilize all of these nutrients from our foods, ultimately nourishing our organs, our brain and each cell. Enzymes are an essential component to a healthy diet.

Anti-Aging Strategies for Your Mind and Emotions

These are essentials for every diet; water, fat, protein, carbohydrates, proper supplementation, probiotics and enzymes. When our bodies consume the correct nutrients and we are able to assimilate the correct nutrients, both our mind and our body are going to be nourished.

When we lack essential nutrients then we are not encouraging feelings of well-being and harmony. An uneasy feeling, a disconnection from the universe develops. This disconnection from others and from ourselves grows, eroding our quality of life. The nutrient deficient mind interferes with our pursuit of enlightenment, awareness and spiritual growth, leaving us feeling tired, lethargic and just plain old. Our mind seems dull and we may suffer from brain fog. That mental clarity and sharpness eludes us.

If I start feeling dull, out of sorts or lethargic, I immediately drink a glass of water. You may not feel thirsty, but dehydration is a common problem. Common symptoms are hunger, impaired memory or concentration, irritability and headaches. I may need a small snack. Once I am sure that my nutritional needs are met, I look further.

When I think about developing a diet for our mind and our emotions it is not one dimensional. It is not just what I put in my mouth. It is important to consider other factors as well. I ask myself the following questions:

Do I need to breathe deeply?
Do I need to take a nap and rejuvenate?
Do I need to meditate?
Do I need to exercise?
Are the thoughts I am thinking serving me?
What is my self-talk?
What type of television shows have I been watching?
What type of movies have I been watching?

What type of music have I been listening to?
Do these things help nurture my mind?
Do these things help nurture my emotions?
Am I cultivating positive feelings and emotions?

Some of my daily practices include listening to audio books while I am driving my car or cleaning my home. Practicing yoga and meditation. Cultivating supportive friendships. Using aromatherapy. Preparing delicious, fresh meals. Learning something new.

I have found that these anti-aging strategies will enhance your life across the board. You will benefit from them, regardless of what diet you subscribe to, whether it is a paleo diet, a vegan or vegetarian diet, Mediterranean diet, any other type of diet out there. Eliminating the toxins and nourishing the body, mind and emotions are essential to maintaining a youthful appearance and youthful spirit. These principles are the foundation to slowing or reversing the aging process and are easily incorporated into any diet.

Lessons Learned

- The basics for every diet include water, quality fats, protein, carbohydrates, fiber, probiotics and enzymes.
- The gut is the second brain; nourish your gut flora by eating a proper, balanced diet.

Action Items

- Eliminate bad fats from you diet as they lead to cellular toxicity.
- Look at the supplements you are taking. Are they made from coal-tar derivatives? Purchase only from a professional line. www.Anti-AgingBody.com

Exercise

I hope this Chapter has caused you to think about the basics to incorporate into your daily living, whether they come from food, drink, emotions or your environment. Pick one thing a week to work on, so it becomes a part of your daily routine. For example, Week 1, you may want to start drinking more water. Week 2 you may want to incorporate breathing exercises into your daily regimen, etc.

CHAPTER SEVEN

The Emotion/Food Connection

"If the head and the body are to be well you need to begin by curing the soul."

Plato

"There is no illness of the body apart from the mind."

Socrates

What did the greatest thinkers of history know? Great thinkers like Plato and Socrates? They knew that there is a direct connection between your emotions and your health. Designing your Anti-Aging Body would be incomplete if it did not include methods to address the emotional aspect of the human experience. Studies have shown that too much stress is so toxic to us that it causes a detrimental chemical impact on our bodies.

It is interesting to note, deaths from heart attacks follow a predictable pattern during the week. They occur at their lowest rate on weekends and significantly jump up on Mondays. Migraines in children are more likely to occur on Monday mornings. It is thought that the reason is due to Monday morning stress - returning to work and school.

Stress Depletes Essential Anti-Aging Nutrients

Stress triggers that fight or flight response that we have all heard about. That fight or flight response sets off a cascade of physiological reactions in our bodies. The body gets the signal that there is danger afoot. The adrenal glands respond by producing stress hormones: adrenaline, cortisol and norepinephrin. Blood rushes away from our digestive organs so we can run from that proverbial tiger. Digestion is unable to function optimally - our meals are not broken down and we are not able to utilize the nutrients we consumed. Symptoms of acid reflux, bloating and gas may appear. Because the entire digestive system is not working properly, elimination is compromised.

The end result may be different for every person. It may manifest as the inability to lose weight or handle cravings. Symptoms of stress are so varied they may result in diabetes, depression, high blood pressure, high cholesterol, hot flashes, low libido and insomnia.

In short, stress causes systemic, chronic inflammation. Inflammation that accelerates aging. Stress squanders our anti-oxidant reserves, most notably vitamins C and E. It depletes all vitamins and minerals that are essential to supporting the liver's detoxification process, including glutathione levels. As I discussed previously, glutathione is a critical nutrient that our liver requires in order to detoxify our bodies and ensure our hormone levels are in balance. If our liver does not have the proper nutrients it is not going to have the ability to detox the body from the toxic substances we ingest on a daily basis. That is why it is critical that we address the stress in our daily lives.

Stress comes from our hectic lifestyles, deadlines, lack of exercise, our diets and our emotions. Let's look at the connection between our emotions and our organs.

Let's look at the connection between our emotions and our organs.

Traditional Chinese Medicine - The Emotion/Organ Connection

Traditional Chinese Medicine Chart

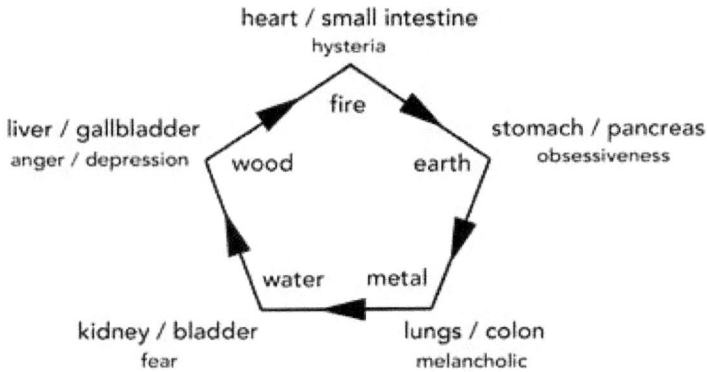

heart / small intestine
hysteria

fire

liver / gallbladder
anger / depression

wood

earth

stomach / pancreas
obsessiveness

water   metal

kidney / bladder
fear

lungs / colon
melancholic

What have the Chinese known for centuries? They know there is a definite connection between certain organs and emotions. For example, in Traditional Chinese Medicine the liver is associated with the emotion of anger. If you are angry or have a lot of unresolved anger, you will have a tendency to have liver issues. The anger will impact the liver and the emotion will lodge there until it is dealt with.

It may manifest as a congested, sluggish liver where you are not detoxifying efficiently or it could manifest more severely. I advise my clients to approach the issue from both directions - emotionally and physically. Address the unresolved anger while nutritionally supporting your liver and possibly doing a liver flush. The liver flush helps to flush those toxic emotions from your body and your soul.

Candice was a 60 year old single woman. She was frustrated that she could not lose weight, couldn't find a life partner and generally unhappy with life. She worked hard on the comprehensive program we designed for her. One component of her program consisted of a colon cleanse and liver flush. She was amazed at the emotions that were released during that process, especially her anger that she tried to keep hidden. In releasing the anger and resentments that had built up over her lifetime, she was able to lose the weight, her skin and eyes were bright and vibrant. She looked at least 10 years younger!

Following this Anti-Aging Body philosophy, I had her keep a journal during the cleanse, writing out the emotions that surfaced. She took the time to address, acknowledge and release those old emotions. She felt an incredible weight had been lifted off of her shoulders and felt years younger.

Kidneys and bladder are associated with fear. It is wise to support your kidneys in the same way. Cleansing that supports and detoxifies your kidneys helps alleviate the fear, while addressing the unresolved fear on an emotional level.

The lungs are associated with grief and the colon is associated with holding onto emotional baggage. A lot of people hold onto resentments, grudges, and negative emotion. Learning to clear your old emotional baggage will accelerate the body's healing process. Keeping a journal while you cleanse is an essential tool in helping to release trapped emotional baggage.

Another client, Donna, discovered she had colon cancer. She used an integrative approach to addressing her health crisis. She received traditional treatment, but attributes her healing to releasing the deep emotional baggage she had been holding onto since she was a small child.

Unfortunately, I find that people don't appreciate the impact their emotions have on their health. Holding on to past hurts and resentments causes current stress and wreaks havoc in our present day lives. Supporting our organs nutritionally and emotionally brings a renewed outlook on life.

Detoxify Your Emotions for a Younger You

Dr. David Hawkins, author Power verses Force, the Hidden Determents of Human Behavior, spent years of his life researching and calibrating human emotion. He discovered that enlightenment calibrated as the highest vibration emotion known. (Refer to the chart found in Chapter 3.) That state of enlightenment that encompasses love, peace, joy, and courage. An ability to move through life with grace, feeling happy and youthful?

In his research, he divided emotions into two categories: power verses force. The highest vibration is enlightenment; below that are peace, joy, love, reason, acceptance, willingness, neutrality and courage. With regard to force, the lowest vibration emotion is shame; then up the scale is guilt, apathy, grief, fear, desire, anger and pride.

How many of us live in shame? We shame ourselves and we shame others. It is these hidden emotions that we do not want anybody to see. We push them down and we do not want to feel them. They are uncomfortable; they are painful. We deceive ourselves into believing that maybe if we deny them, they will go away. But they don't. The way out of this is not to push down these emotions and deny them, but to acknowledge and feel them. Allow them to alchemize into something beautiful that you can use your experiences to create with and to serve others. You have these uncomfortable emotions because you have attached a meaning to an event that happened in your life.

Dr. Wayne Dyer tells a story of his childhood. He is father abandoned him and his brothers when he was a very young child. His mother put him in foster homes until he was the age of 10. He had a choice. Become bitter, resentful and angry - or attach an empowering meaning to his childhood. After working through the emotions, he realized that his childhood could be no other way. He needed to learn self-reliance at an early age. He changed the meaning he attached to those events.

Keep in mind, nothing has meaning except for the meaning you give it. For example, if there is a watch that you like in the store, there is little to no emotional attachment to it. However, if the love of your life saved up their money, knew you would appreciate it and gave it to you for your anniversary, it would take on a new meaning. It would have sentimental value. It is the same watch, but you attached and empowering meaning to it.

It is the same with circumstances we encounter. There have been many times that someone has hurt my feelings. I attached a meaning to my friend's actions. If I am feeling down, I may tell myself that they don't value our relationship as I do, or I may tell myself that they are selfish. If I am honest with myself, I find that the meaning I attach to an event is related to my level of stress. If I am feeling grateful and appreciative about life, the same behavior by my friend would be met with compassion and concern.

Let me illustrate. For example, if you are to meet a friend for lunch and they cancel on you at the last minute, do you get angry and tell yourself that your friend is inconsiderate, selfish and they don't care for you? Or do you tell yourself that your friend probably had a good reason and would not intentionally do something to hurt you?

I know that may seem to be a silly example, however I have had a friend get really angry with me when I had to cancel a lunch. She had suffered unnecessary heartache and pain because she assumed that my actions came from a selfish intent. Only later did she come to find out that it was a complete misunderstanding and our friendship was restored. The events were the same. It was only the meaning she attached to the situation that changed. She could have been experiencing love for me and herself instead of suffering. Commonly, it is the cumulative effect of these little irritations that compound and have a detrimental effect on our quality of life.

It is time to take an inventory of our lives and look at the meanings we have attach to the circumstances. One of my friend's said to me one day "We make up these stories in our head every day, why not make up a story that serves you?"

The way out of this swamp land of negative emotions is to address these emotions and expose them to the light. It takes courage to work through unpleasant emotions but the reward is that we will gain access to all of our emotions and move up the scale toward love, joy, peace and enlightenment. The great news is that you do not need to be the victim of your emotions. Our emotions add beauty and texture to our lives - yes, even the unpleasant ones. The hurtful emotions we have buried within us tend to rise up, rearing their ugly heads at the most inopportune times. We fight and struggle to deny them. This internal battle takes a toll on us, physically and emotionally. When these emotions leak out, a common response is to shame ourselves or even blame others. We see these emotions as inconsistent with how we perceive ourselves or how we want others to perceive us. There is no emotional freedom or enlightenment without addressing the emotions that have been controlling us.

It has been difficult, but I have learned to welcome those feelings as signals, showing me the way to a happier, freer life. I can transform and alleviate the stress in my life. There is no enlightenment without addressing the emotions that have been controlling us.

Lessons Learned

- Our emotions directly affect us physically and spiritually.
- Stress depletes nutrients that are essential for anti-aging and detoxification.

Action Items

- Address the stress in your life. Is the stressor really worth the damage to your health?
- When you feel down, look at the meaning you are attributing to that situation. Can you change your perspective and give it an empowering meaning?

Exercise

I hope this chapter has caused you to think about how stress impacts your daily life. Pick one thing a week to work on, so it becomes a part of your daily routine. For example, Week 1, you may want to take an inventory of what the sources of stress (i.e. work stress, home stress, relationship stress, etc.). Week 2 you may want to carve out time to start to meditate each morning, etc.

CHAPTER EIGHT

Body Toxins

"Food, one assumes, provides nourishment; but Americans eat it fully aware that small amounts of poison have been added to improve its appearance and delay its putrefaction."

John Cage

We can't escape from exposure to toxins. They are just a part of living nowadays. We can, however eliminate some of the most common neurotoxins that we are exposed to day-in, day-out. It is unrealistic to run off to a mountain top to attempt to live a life of complete purity. Not only that, it would not be very fun. The solution is to design a lifestyle that protects us from common everyday exposure to toxins.

It is a given that every day we are exposed to toxins from all sorts of sources. They are absorbed orally, via inhalation, transdermally through your skin. Skin is our largest organ. Our skin acts as a sponge, absorbing everything we put on it. Why is it that we think we can wash our skin with antibacterial soaps and those chemicals won't be directly absorbed into our blood stream affecting us? Why do we think that antibacterial soaps will only kill the bad bacteria and not the necessary, beneficial bacteria? It just doesn't work that way.

We can't get rid of every toxin out there, but we can take huge strides in eliminating the worst of the worst from our environment: neurotoxins, pesticides and dietary toxins.

Fluoride Ages You

One of the most insidious toxins that we are exposed to on a daily basis is fluoride. It is a neurotoxin. Neurotoxins are specifically designed to target the nervous system and damage it by disrupting the signaling that allows neurons to communicate with each other. We are exposed to fluoride from our toothpaste, from our mouthwash, we get it when we go to the dentist and have our teeth cleaned. There are fluoride rinses and they even have fluoride vitamins for children.

If that wasn't bad enough, our government has deemed this neurotoxin essential to our health and has put it directly into our drinking water. This is something we consume unknowingly on a daily basis. We drink water, wash our vegetables, make tea and coffee with fluoride laden water. This is crazy! Fluoride is a neurotoxin.

The history of fluoride and how it has been incorporated into our daily lives is really frightening but is also fascinating. Hitler realized its toxicity and used fluoride to dumb down the population. It is an industrial waste product of aluminum manufacturing, as well as a waste product of the nuclear and fertilizer industries. It is the main active ingredient in some pesticides and rat poison.

I used to think that fluoride came from a sanitary lab, then placed in our drinking water. Nothing could be further from the truth. As I stated, it is an industrial waste product that, without being processed or sanitized, comes from the factory and is dumped into the water supply. This is scary; this is what we are giving our children. If you have a baby that is fed formula they can be consuming fluoride in toxic levels. Fluoridated water is used when food manufacturers make their sodas, energy drinks, and bottled teas. The public is consuming fluoride from all sorts of different sources.

Fluoride can lead to crippling skeletal fluorosis. It also leads to increased lead absorption and lead is a neurotoxin in its own right. It can lead to genetic damage and cell death; it can cause brain damage and lower your IQ which of course does nothing to help us in keeping our minds youthful and alert. It impairs thyroid function, is a contributing factor in dementia and it inactivates enzymes. There are no health benefits to fluoride, despite what the American Dental Association has been promoting for nearly 70 years.

Fluoride is attracted to our pineal gland and the pineal gland is a portal to spirituality and higher consciousness. It is located at the point of the sixth chakra or the third eye and it is vital to intuition. MRI's have been on done the pineal gland of subjects of all ages. It was discovered that in both adults and even in young children that the pineal gland was calcified to varying degrees. Autopsies have proven that it is the fluoride that is being attracted to the pineal gland.

The calcification of the pineal gland was first recognized and brought to light by a study in 1990 by Dr. Jennifer Luke. Dr. Luke's research determined that the pineal gland, even in young adults, will be calcified to some degree. Research has demonstrated that everyone to some degree, by the time they reach adulthood has a calcified pineal gland.

When considering the subject of anti-aging, the pineal gland is of paramount importance. It is the gland that synthesizes and secrets melatonin which regulates your circadian rhythms and your sleep cycle. It also regulates the onset of puberty. It helps protect the body from cell damage and free radical damage. The pineal gland may be small in size, but it is a powerhouse in reversing or slowing the aging process.

This may be a small gland but its importance cannot be underestimated. For that reason, it is essential to implement a lifestyle that is aimed at decalcifying the pineal gland. Sunshine is something that helps to decalcify the pineal gland. Other practices include sun gazing, meditation, getting adequate rest and of course eating the proper foods.

There is an old Ayurvedic remedy for decalcifying the pineal gland. It consists of blending three ingredients, shilajit which is a mineral supplement that is very high in fulvic acid; ghee, which is clarified butter, and raw honey. According to Ayurvedic tradition, if you take this on a consistent basis it helps to decalcify the pineal gland.

A few other foods that can help to decalcify the pineal gland are raw cacao, goji berries, cilantro, watermelon, coconut oil, hemp seeds, seaweed and noni juice. Meditation will stimulate the decalcification of the pineal gland. A great way to further accelerate the decalcification process is to use good essential oils like lavender, frankincense and sandalwood while you meditate. These oils can be put in a diffuser or nebulizer. When they are inhaled, they immediately cross the blood brain barrier and directly impact the limbic system of the brain. When added to bath water, they are absorbed directly through the skin.

I also recommend incorporating raw apple cider vinegar into your daily regimen. You can put about eight tablespoons of the Braggs apple cider vinegar into a quart of drinking water and drink that throughout the day.

Fluoride's damage on the body is far and wide. It interferes with the thyroid hormone conversion from T4 to the active T3; it attaches to the iodine receptors preventing iodine from working.

In summary, there is absolutely no medicinal value to fluoride exposure. It only serves to impair your health, vitality and intuition. So, lets start by throwing out that toothpaste and mouthwash and get a good water filter.

Chlorine Ages You

Another toxin most of us are exposed to on a daily basis is chlorine. Per the CDC's own website chlorine is a potential agent for chemical terrorism. It is used in pesticides and solvents. It kills bacteria, both good and bad. No doubt this will have a detrimental effect on your gut flora.

In World War I it was used as a choking agent and as of now there is no antidote for chlorine exposure. As with fluoride, chlorine interferes with thyroids conversation of the thyroid hormone T4 to the active T3. It attaches to the iodine receptors preventing iodine from attaching and from doing its work in the thyroid gland.

As with fluoride, we are exposed to chlorine every day. When we take that nice hot shower, the chlorine vaporizes and we inhale it. So along with inhaling the vaporized chlorine, our skin is acting like a sponge, absorbing the chlorine. It is in detergents and in cleaning products that are used in nearly every room in our homes.

It seems we can't escape it. Chlorine is all around us. Look at your cleaning products and detergents and determine what you are using around your home.

There are non-chlorine alternatives available to us. One of the easiest and most inexpensive ways to protect ourselves from the chlorine assault is to install a shower filter.

Bromine Ages You

Bromine is another toxic element that is all around us. Being exposed to this toxin will directly impair your health and quest for the mental clarity and youthfulness. It builds up in your central nervous system and it is a depressant. It can trigger central nervous system and respiratory failure as well as paranoia and psychotic symptoms.

So what is bromine, anyway? Do you remember back to your chemistry class and the periodic table? Bromine is an element found on the periodic table from the halide family. Other halides include fluorine and chlorine, which we have already discussed. Bromine's uses are wide and varied. It is the active ingredient in potassium bromate, a dough conditioner. It is used in pesticides, plastics, baked goods, soft drinks, medication, pool treatments and it is also used in fire retardants. How could something so heavily used in our food supply be dangerous if it is allowed by the FDA? The FDA seems to be turning a blind eye to its health risks.

It is an endocrine disruptor, which will wreak havoc on your hormones. Bromine is also the active ingredient in methyl bromide, a pesticide. This is what is heavily sprayed on conventionally grown strawberries. In fact, our conventionally grown strawberries are saturated with methyl bromide throughout their entire growing season.

The growers want to make sure that the strawberries are not going to be eaten by pests before they are sold to us. Strawberries are like sponges, absorbing whatever chemicals are sprayed on them. This is one food that should never be eaten, even those tempting chocolate dipped strawberries, unless they are organic. Otherwise, you will become a sponge as well, soaking up all those neurotoxic chemicals from the strawberry.

Unfortunately, the use of bromine does not stop at flour conditioners and pesticides. There a myriad of other dietary sources of bromine. BVO, which is brominated vegetable oil, is added to citrus drinks because it suspends the citrus flavor in the liquid. This is commonly found in sodas.

For example, if you drink Mountain Dew you will be drinking brominated vegetable oil. It is in other citrus drinks as well.

Bromine poses such a significant health risk that the UK, Canada and Brazil have banned it in breads. The only way to insure that your foods are safe from its toxic effects is to go on an organic diet.

Cumulative Effect of Toxins Causes Accelerated Aging

I am sure you have heard of the magic of the compounding principle. It is typically referred to when discussing investments. It is where the cumulative effects of adding small amounts of money to an investment over time, results in large nest egg in the end. Increasing the frequency of compounding dramatically increases the value of the investment.

This principle is great and works to your advantage when you are talking about money. However, the same principle applies to the cumulative effect of toxins on our bodies. Low exposure multiple times a day, over an extended amount of time, leads to a huge toxic overload. The FDA passes on these toxins, declaring them GRAS (Generally Regarded As Safe) since they occur in such small doses. Their philosophy seems to be no harm, no foul. The problem with that logic is there are innumerable chemicals, additives and dyes in our food supply and environment, that we are being exposed to on a daily basis in so-called "safe" levels. The insanity of this "logic" is that the exposure adds up over time and no one has ever tested the interaction of the "safe levels" of these individual chemicals when they are combined!

Chances are, you are not just drinking the brominated vegetable oil that is in your citrus drink. It is likely made with fluoridated, chlorinated water which was drunk after taking a shower with chlorinated water and brushing your teeth with fluoride toothpaste.

Not to mention the myriad other chemical-laden personal body care products typically used, like deodorant, moisturizer and make-up. All of these toxins build up, taxing our bodies, causing premature aging.

Is It a Health Food or Does It Cause Premature Aging?

Another class of toxins I would like to touch on are dietary toxins. These are foods we are exposed to on a daily basis and sometimes passed off as "health" foods. My short list of the most common unhealthy "health" foods include gluten, dairy, soy and agave nectar.

Gluten Accelerates Aging

Looking at the food pyramid that our government promoted up until about 2011, it was recommended that a healthy diet consist of 6 - 11 servings of whole grain per day. The food pyramid has been replaced by "MyPlate" which recommends 30% of your diet consist of whole grains, such as toast, cereal or pasta.

These grains are primarily made from glutenous grains, such as wheat, rye and barely. Gluten is considered a staple. Entire meals are planned around gluten. Sandwiches, pizza and beer, pasta, cakes and cookies all contain gluten. Many people eat bread or pasta at every meal!

Gluten is found in sauces, including soy sauce. It is used as a thickener in soups. It is in most desserts. It is used in spices so they don't clump together. If you order grilled fish, it is likely that the cook coated it with a fine layer of flour to keep the fish from sticking to the grill. The list of uses for gluten is nearly endless.

Gluten not only affects those with the autoimmune condition of Celiac's disease; it affects those with Non-Celiac Gluten sensitivity (NCGS), causing gut permeability which can lead a whole host of other autoimmune disorders, from Hashimoto's disease to rheumatoid arthritis. More people are affected by NCGS than Celiac's disease. The symptoms for NCGS are far and wide, and not necessarily tied to digestive issues. This means that those individuals who suffer from NCGS will unknowingly be causing damage to their bodies by continuing to eat gluten.

Soy Accelerates Aging

I acknowledge that soy is a very controversial subject. I am not a soy advocate. Soy has been heavily promoted as a health food, especially to women. It is not a health food by any stretch of the imagination, in fact, it is an anti-nutrient. It is estrogenic, meaning it is an endocrine disruptor. Most of it is genetically modified and it is toxic if it is consumed raw. Soy impedes the sexual maturation of boys and it accelerates it in girls. It can cause digestive problems and has been linked to some cancers. It is best to completely leave soy out of your diet due to the detrimental affect it will have on your health.

Many people point to studies that show that Japanese women have lower incidences of certain cancers. However, I would like to point out that their diets are not the same as the SAD. Their diets consists of large quantities of fresh vegetables. Further, most of the soy they consume is non-GMO and fermented. Just looking at the headline of a study does not tell the entire story.

Soy is not a life-enhancing food for your body. Given that soy consumption can lead to cognitive decline, it certainly is not a food that will help slow or reverse the aging of your brain. Anything that is going to impact your brain in that manner, anything that will result in the decline of your health will prevent you from developing your healthy, vibrant and youthful life. An excellent book on this topic is "The Whole Soy Story: The Dark Side of America's Favorite Health Food" by Kaayla Daniel.

Agave Nectar Accelerates Aging

Agave nectar is another food that was heavily promoted as a health food: many people in health and wellness field jumped on the bandwagon and promoted agave nectar as a great sweetener. The reason it has been promoted as a health food is that it is relatively low on the glycemic index.

A low glycemic food does not spike your blood sugar. Diabetics and those concerned about their blood sugar levels will use agave rather than sugar, thinking they are doing right by their body.

However, the body process agave in the same way as high fructose corn syrup is processed in the body, going straight to the liver for metabolism. It does have a low glycemic index which means that it won't cause blood sugar spikes. However, its affects can be much worse. It is toxic to the body in that it elevates the triglyceride levels.

Organic verses Conventional - Take the Burden Off Your Body

When we are looking at the toxins we are exposed to on a daily basis it is of critical importance to consume organic. I know people don't want to spend more money for organic products. I have heard the argument that the nutrient content is the same; there is no difference between organic and conventional. I disagree with their opinion. The science backs up the fact that organic produce is more nutrient dense than conventionally grown produce. However, I personally do not even engage in that debate.

In conventional farming, the soil is fumigated with neurotoxic chemicals, killing all beneficial bacteria. The crops are sprayed with neurotoxic herbicides and pesticides. The soil is depleted necessitating the use of fertilizers. Most of these fertilizers are petroleum based. Some fertilizers come from manure lagoons that are found on industrial factory livestock farms. They spray this untreated animal waste directly on crops, increasing the risk of salmonella contamination.

If that were not bad enough, some crops are genetically modified. Conventionally grown produce may look beautiful, but it is laden with toxic petroleum based chemicals.

With organically grown produce, farmers focus on growing healthy soil. If the soil full of healthy microbes, if the soil nutrient rich, the outcome is healthy, strong plants. It is the terrain that matters.

An easy way to determine whether or not you are purchasing organic produce is to look at the little sticker grocery store placed on it. If the sticker starts with a 4 and it is four digits it is conventionally grown. If the little sticker starts with a 9 and it is five digits then it is organic. Refer to my website www.Anti-AgingBody.com for further information regarding organics.

Dairy - Does It Do a Body Good?

There is a huge debate over the health benefits of dairy products, especially milk. I believe milk does not do a body good, despite the dairy industry spending billions of advertising dollars telling you otherwise. At least not the homogenized, pasteurized milk sold in the grocery stores.

Pasteurization heats the milk up in order to kill any possible bacteria or pathogens. Pasteurized milk is "dead," and offers little in terms of real nutritional value to anyone. Enzymes are destroyed and vitamins (such as A, C, B-6 and B-12) are diminished, while interfering with vitamin D absorption.

Homogenization also involves high temperatures, but the purpose is to make the fat globules smaller so they are evenly dispersed throughout the milk. During the pasteurization and homogenization processes the fragile milk proteins are radically transformed stripping them from possessing any health enhancing properties to proteins that can actually worsen your health.

Cows are pumped up with hormones and antibiotics. They undergo annual cycles of artificial insemination, pregnancy and birth. They are milked for about 10 months out of the year. This simply is not sustainable. These cows are only productive for about 2 years. Their udders become infected, causing the milk to contain pus and blood. According to the USDA, 1 in 6 dairy cows suffer from clinical mastitis (udder infections).

If you do decide to incorporate dairy into your diet, make sure it is organic. Organic dairies are held to a higher standard of cleanliness and better treatment of the animals. A little research into the treatment of dairy cows and the quality of milk produced by these non-organic dairies will definitely persuade you to consume organic dairy, if you choose to consume dairy at all.

Lessons Learned

- Being exposed to toxins is inevitable, but we can eliminate some of the most dangerous toxins by limiting our exposure to fluoride, chlorine and bromine.
- Small, daily toxic exposure accumulates in our body, causing cumulative damage over time.

Action Items

- Buy organic as much as possible.
- Find dairy alternatives, as dairy consumption does not have any real nutritional value.

Exercise

I hope this chapter has caused you to think about the body toxins you are exposed to in your daily life. Pick one thing a week to work on, so it becomes a part of your daily routine. For example, Week 1, you may want to make a commitment to purchase only organic produce. Week 2 you may want to make a commitment to eliminate dairy, etc.

Follow this link to download the 60-Day Anti-Aging Body Master Plan worksheet to help you track and create your personalized Master Plan. By writing out your thoughts and ideas, you will be designing your blueprint for success!

http://goo.gl/E5FFMj

CHAPTER NINE

Exercise

_____

"If we could give every individual the right amount of nourishment and exercise, not too little and not too much, we would have found the safest way to health."

Hippocrates

Exercise - An Essential Component to Your Anti-Aging Body

Exercise is essential to developing an Anti-Aging Body. When contemplating designing your Anti-Aging Body protocol, incorporating consistent, moderate exercise is a key component. Exercise provides powerful benefits to the physical body as well as the soul and spirit. It strengthens us while at the same time can serve to detoxify us, physically, mentally and emotionally.

Regarding the physical body, when you start huffing and puffing, and breathing deeply, you are using more of your lungs. Your lungs are an organ of elimination. They eliminate CO_2 and toxins. This helps to alkalinize your body.

Exercise also helps with your lymph flow. Lymph plays a key role in the immune system. It consists of clear, watery fluid that circulates through the body removing bacteria and proteins from the tissues, cleansing us on a cellular level. Basically, it is designed to keep the body clean. I think of it as the sewage system of the body. And, nobody wants a backed-up sewage system!

It is interesting to note that there is more lymph in your body than there is blood. Your blood, however, has the heart to pump it through the body. The lymph system does not have a pump; however, it is vital to keep the lymph from stagnating. Keeping in mind the function and design of the lymph system, it is easy to see that the body was constructed to exercise on a daily basis. The flow of your lymph is dependent upon movement: Movement from the diaphragm and movement from exercise such as rebounding.

Deep breathing will cause the diaphragm to expand and contract, causing the lymph to flow. Most people are chest breathers rather than belly breathers. It is important to focus on breathing deeply, from your belly to fully activate your diaphragm.

Rebounding uses gravitational pressure to activate the lymph system. Rebounding is accomplished by jumping up and down on a mini-trampoline. This is one of the most effective methods of stimulating lymph flow because it actually exercises every cell of the body on a cellular level, ensuring that each cell is able to rid itself of its metabolic waste. Even though rebounding is excellent for stimulating lymph flow, walking is superb as well! In fact, it is imperative that you just get off that couch and start moving. Find an activity that you enjoy - and do it!

The benefits of exercise extend past your physical body to enhancing your brain and mind. Exercise boosts the neurotransmitter production of the brain, which directly improves mood.

Studies have demonstrated that on a long-term basis, exercise is more effective in alleviating depression than medication. The Mayo Clinic published studies that demonstrated that exercise eases depression by releasing "feel-good" brain chemicals (endorphins), reducing immune system chemicals that can exacerbate depression and increase body temperature, which tends to have calming effects.

A Harvard study published in 2005 found that walking fast for about 35 minutes a day five times a week or 60 minutes a day three times a week had a significant influence on mild to moderate depression symptoms. It was also determined that walking fast for only 15 minutes a day five times a week or doing stretching exercises three times a week did not help as much.

What does all of this mean to you? The bottom line is that exercise enhances the release of endorphins, improves natural immunity and reduces the perception of pain and serves to improve mood.

The body will find its own natural balance of neurotransmitters and the end result will be elevated moods and better sleep.

Aside from releasing endorphins and elevating your mood, additional mental benefits of exercise are accomplished when your body composition starts to change. When your lean body mass starts to increase and your body fat decreases, insulin sensitivity increases. Increased insulin sensitivity results in increased brain health, as discussed earlier.

Clearly there exists a symbiotic relationship between the body and the spirit. What is designed to help and heal the body will also help and heal the mind.

Yoga

I am particularly fond of yoga because I have witnessed it's practice transform lives. Its poses can activate the lymphatic system, help regulate the thyroid, improve metabolism and aid in sleep. It is an ideal integrative practice as it seeks to strengthen body, soul and spirit through exercise, breathing and nutrition. It becomes a way of living, harmonizing your interpersonal life with our chaotic world. Yoga seeks to incorporate virtues such as integrity, compassion, patience, humility and non-attachment into your daily life and in practical ways.

There is a Sanskrit word, drishti. It has many meanings, however what resonates most with me is the idea that it is the practice of gazing outward while bringing the focus inward. I use this concept in my daily life. I focus outward on what I would like to accomplish in my day or in my life, while at the same time focusing inward on who I need to become in order to accomplish my goals. This one practice helps to center me and keep me balanced.

Lessons Learned

- Your lungs are an organ of elimination, and when you exercise you are using more of your lungs and detoxifying your body.
- Exercise is more effective in addressing depression than medication.

Action Items

- Integrate exercise into your daily activity.
- Decide what is your Drishti? Focus on that, while focusing on who you need to become.

Exercise

I hope this Chapter has caused you to think about exercise. Pick one thing a week to work on, so it becomes a part of your daily routine. For example, if you do not exercise regularly, Week 1, you may want to start walking, making a commitment to walk for 30 minutes a day. Week 2 you may want to branch out and try a different type of exercise (i.e. yoga, stretching, cardio). Find something you enjoy, and have fun!

Follow this link to download the 60-Day Anti-Aging Body Master Plan worksheet to help you track and create your personalized Master Plan. By writing out your thoughts and ideas, you will be designing your blueprint for success!

http://goo.gl/E5FFMj

CHAPTER TEN

Recipes and Rituals

"Grace isn't a little prayer you chant before receiving a meal. It's a way to live."

~Attributed to Jacqueline Winspear

Eating is a Fun Way to Reverse Aging

I love to eat. I eat every two to three hours. I think it is fun and delicious. Eating is one of the simple delights of life. I love to feel good. I have made such a strong emotional connection between eating well and feeling good that the two are forever linked. I love the way I feel when I eat a fresh salad, piled high with fresh, organic veggies. I feel light, sexy and youthful!

I love my chocolate. Raw cacao is full of life-enhancing, age-reversing anti-oxidants and minerals. I have designed an Anti-Aging Body lifestyle that works for me.

I realize that there is more to eating, than just filling my belly. I incorporate eating rituals to fill my soul as well.

Eating Rituals

When I sit down with a meal, I think about what I am about to eat, I think about the source, I think about this food and realize it is going to become me. To me, there is nothing more intimate nor more spiritual than eating because this substance becomes me; this becomes who I am as a person. This meal influences my thoughts and emotions. This meal that I have before me can either bring health and vitality or it can bring me down and bring me disease and sickness.

Looking at my meal before me, I take a moment to express gratitude for it. When I prepare a meal, I think about my family and friends I will be serving. I look at this mealtime as an opportunity to bond with others, with my family, with nature and even bond with myself.

I pause and take a breath rather than diving right in and eating. I ask my clients to take a moment to pray, and express gratitude for the meal before them. If they eating something that is not the best, for example, a bag of chips, accept it with gratitude. Don't stress over it. Don't beat yourself up and feel guilty. As we have discussed, those emotions can be just as toxic. Accept it with gratitude and let it go and get back on track.

I also advise my client to assess where they are in their journey of reversing the ravages of aging. I challenge them to decide on one area to improve upon and master that one thing. It does not matter what that one new thing is - whether it is learning a new recipe, cutting out soda or learn a new breathing exercise. Implement that into your lifestyle, and step by step upgrade your lifestyle. Adapt that one practice in a manner that will work with your lifestyle. Unless you are facing a health challenge or are extremely motivated, I have found that trying to make too many changes at one time can result in no long term changes being made.

If you are ready to take your life to the next level and incorporate some Anti-Aging Body strategies, it is a good idea to have some basic kitchen tools. It will make upgrading your lifestyle easier.

Tools of the Trade-The Necessary Kitchen Gear

Let's take a look at some of the basic tools that you will need in your kitchen.

1. **Knives** - A good, sharp, and well cared for knife is a must. I prefer ceramic knives because they are sharper, lightweight,

easy to clean, and leave no metallic taste or smell. For cracking open those coconuts, you will need something a bit more substantial than a ceramic knife!

2. **Blenders** - A strong blender is essential for making all those delicious smoothies, sauces, and puddings. There are many blenders out there and must do your research before going out and purchasing one. I would highly recommend investing in the right blender. A strong blender can make a huge difference. My favorite is K-Tec, as it has a 10 year warranty and can easily sit on your countertop.

3. **Food Processors** - I use the Omega brand as it comes with a great warranty.

4. **Juicers** - Given the wide variety of juicers, figuring out which one to purchase can be daunting! Just like the blender one must do the research. Different juicers to different things. There are citrus juicers, masticating juicers and centrifugal juicer, to name a few. I use the Omega VRT360. I like this juicer because I think that it is one of the most versatile and easiest to clean. It is great for juicing and for making nut milks.

Recipes Tips

I design my meals to support my body's needs. I know that the cause of dis-ease boils down to toxicity and deficiency. If my body is toxic, symptoms will begin to appear. If I don't get the nutrients I need, my body and organs will suffer.

It is important to design a meal plan that will aid in the detoxification of your body. The two main organs I focus on are the liver and the bowels. I know that the liver does double duty. It is constantly working. It detoxifies the body, breaks down excess hormones, manufactures bile, among other things. The recipes that follow are designed to give the liver the nutrients it needs so that it can do its job.

To further support your body's detoxification, make sure that your bowels are functioning optimally. It is important to strive to consume a least 25 grams of fiber each day.

The brain and central nervous system are the master control system of your body. They need plenty of high quality raw fats and fresh, spring water.

A tip for making these recipes more nutritious is to make a bone strengthening, immune enhancing or anti-oxidant tea, substituting the tea for the water in any recipe. Simmer any combination of the following herbs: oat straw, horse tail, stinging nettles, he shou wu tea and reishi mushrooms. Get creative and make any tea you desire.

If I am making something with a more fruity flavor, I will make gynostemma or schizandra tea and add that to the recipe rather than water.

Recipes

Smoothies, Juices and Drinks

Glowing Skin Sweet and Sour Smoothie
Ingredients:
2 cups frozen organic strawberries
1 large red bell organic pepper
1 persian cucumber
1 organic lemon
Pinch of cayenne

Directions: Blend all ingredients until smooth. If you want a juice, you can juice all ingredients except for the strawberries. Place the juice in a blender and add the strawberries, blend to desired consistency.

Anti-Oxidant Beauty Smoothie
Ingredients:
2 cups frozen organic strawberries, raspberries or blackberries
1/3 cup raw cauliflower *
1 large organic apple
1 organic lemon

Directions: Blend all ingredients until smooth. If you want a juice, you can juice all ingredients except for the berries. Place the juice in a blender and add the berries, blend to desired consistency.

*Note: Some people cannot consume raw cauliflower as it has a goitrogenic effect on their bodies. If this is the case, eliminate the cauliflower.

Mineral-Rich Green Smoothie (for Liver Support)
Ingredients:
1 cup dandelion
1 cup stinging nettles
1 cup Swiss Chard (any variety)
2 cups fresh, spring water
1 - 2 dates with pits removed

Directions: Blend all ingredients until smooth. If you want a juice, you can juice all ingredients except for the dates. Place the juice in a blender and add the dates, blend to desired consistency.

Green Smoothie with Banana
Ingredients:
1 cup dandelion
1 cup kale (any variety)
1 cup Swiss Chard (any variety)
2 cups fresh, spring water
1 large banana

Directions: Blend all ingredients until smooth. If you want a juice, you can juice all ingredients except for the banana. Place the juice in a blender and add the banana, blend to desired consistency.

Tropical Delight Smoothie (Heavy Metal Chelator)
Ingredients:
1 mango or 1 cup frozen mango
1 handful organic cilantro
1/2 fresh cucumber
2 cups fresh, spring water
1 organic lime

Directions: Blend all ingredients until smooth.
This has a delightful, light flavor that pack a powerful punch against heavy metals.

Low Glycemic Green Juice for Liver Support
Ingredients:
2 cups dandelion
2 cups Swiss Chard (any variety)
1 cucumber
2 - 3 stalks celery
1 large apple

Directions: Juice all ingredients in your Omega VRT360

Omega-3 Raw Chai Smoothie
Ingredients:
2 frozen organic bananas
1 cup walnut milk
1 cup freshly juiced carrot juice
1 teaspoon cinnamon
1 teaspoon vanilla extract
Pinch of sea salt

Directions: Blend all ingredients until smooth.

Radiant Beauty Coconut Smoothie
Ingredients:
1 fresh young thai coconut
1 tbsp raw hemp seeds
1 tbsp raw cacao powder
1 tsp raw maca powder
1 tsp raw mesquite powder
1 handful of ice

Directions: Blend all ingredients until smooth.

Vanilla Nut Milk
Ingredients:
1 cup soaked nuts (choose your favorite or experiment with brazil, almond, hazelnut, walnut, or macadamia nuts, etc)
2 tablespoons coconut butter
4 cups fresh spring water
2 dates, pitted (optional)
1 vanilla bean, scraped (optional)
Pinch of himalayan salt

Directions: Blend all ingredients until smooth. Strain milk through a fine sleeve or nut milk bag. If you have the Omega VRT360 or similar vertical juicer, run the nuts and water through the juicer. Place the nut milk in your blender and add the coconut butter, dates, vanilla and salt. Blend. Refrigerate and enjoy!

Nut milks are great substitutions for water in smoothies. They can be used in cereals and frozen treats.

Make sure to keep the pulp from the nuts as you can dehydrate this and use as flour in other recipes.

Soup, Salad, Sandwiches and More

Cleansing and Fortifying Salad
1/2 cup arugula
1/2 cup watercress
1/4 cup cilantro
1/2 cup baby greens
1/2 red bell pepper
1/2 cucumber
1/2 avocado
1/4 cup walnuts
1/4 cup dehydrated cranberries
1 chopped heirloom tomato

Directions: Wash all ingredients. Chop all ingredients into bite sized pieces. Place in a bowl, toss, mixing thoroughly.

Simple Salad Dressing
Ingredients:
1/2 cup apple cider vinegar
1/3 cup extra-virgin olive oil
1 tsp. Nama Shoyu or Organic Tamari
1 tsp. coconut nectar or raw honey

Directions: Combine all ingredients in a salad dressing bottle and shake vigorously, or blend in blender. I love this recipe because it is basic and simple. This means that you can get creative adding herbs and spices to your liking.

Asparagus Support Your Liver Detox Soup
Ingredients:
10 thick or 25 thin (1 bunch) stalks of steamed asparagus
2/3 cups pecans (soaked) or almond (soaked)
2 cups fresh spring water
2 tbsp. olive oil or avocado oil
3 tbsp. fresh squeezed lemon juice

2 cloves minced garlic
½ tsp Himalayan salt
½ tsp black pepper
½ avocado (cut in chunks)

Directions: Lightly steam asparagus. Add steamed asparagus, soaked and rinsed pecans or almonds, fresh spring water; olive oil or avocado oil, lemon juice, garlic, salt and pepper to blender. Blend one 50 second cycle at speed 10. Serve slightly warm and garnish with avocado chunks in the bowl.

Onion Bread Sandwich
Ingredients:
2 slices of raw, dehydrated onion bread (see below)
2 tbsp. Fresh garden herb pate (see below)
Fresh alfalfa sprouts
1/2 avocado
1/2 tomato

Directions: Spread the pate on both slices of onion bread. Layer sprouts, avocado and tomato and top with the other slice of onion bread.

Onion Bread
Ingredients:
3 large onions, finely chopped
3/4 cup chia seeds
3/4 cup raw, sprouted sunflower seeds
1/2 cup Nama Shoyu
1/3 cup olive oil

Directions: Finely slice and chop the onions. Place the chia seeds, sunflower seeds Nama Shoyu and olive oil in the K-Tec blender or food processor. Mix all ingredients thoroughly. Add the onions by hand. Spread the mixture thinly on teflex sheets. Dehydrate at 100 degrees for approximately 24 hours. Flip the bread onto a tray with mesh only and remove teflex. Dehydrate another 12 hours. Once dehydrated cut into 9 equal pieces

Fresh Garden Herb Pate
Ingredients:
1 tbsp lemon juice
1 cup soaked sunflower seeds
1/2 tsp unpasteurized light chickpea miso
1/2 tsp plus a pinch of sea salt
2 garlic cloves
1/8 cup basil finely chopped
1/2 tsp rosemary finely chopped
1/2 tsp thyme finely chopped
1/2 tsp oregano finely chopped
1/4 tsp sage finely chopped
2/3 cups fresh spring water

Directions: Mince garlic. If using fresh herbs mince them very fine. Blend soaked seeds, lemon juice, salt, minced garlic, miso in blender until mostly smooth (add water). Mix in herbs by hand. This is a delicious pate and a great addition to a dipping platter or as a plate on a veggie sandwich.

Onion Bread Bruschetta
Ingredients:
2 slices of raw, dehydrated onion bread
3 small heirloom tomatoes - chopped
1 clove garlic - finely minced
1/2 Tbsp. extra virgin olive oil
1/2 tsp. balsamic vinegar
3 - 4 fresh basil leaves - finely chopped
Salt and freshly ground pepper to taste
1/2 avocado

Directions: Place the chopped tomatoes, minced garlic, olive oil, vinegar, chopped basil, salt and pepper in a bowl and mix. Place the tomato mixture on both slices of onion bread. Layer the sliced avocado on top. Cut in small pieces. Serve immediately as the bread may become soggy if left to sit too long.

Fermented Vegetables
Ingredients:
Choose raw, organic vegetables of choice: cabbage, celery, sweet potatoes, carrots, or beets. Get creative and use your favorite vegetables.
Himalayan salt
Fresh spring water
Mason jars

Directions: Chop your favorite organic, raw vegetables. Place them in a large bowl and submerge them in just enough fresh, spring water to cover the vegetables; add a handful of salt, mixing thoroughly. Stuff the mason jars with the vegetables and water. Top off the jar with a cabbage leaf, making sure all air is out of the jar. Place the jar on the counter for 6 to 7 days. If you like, you can also use a starter mix, although this is not necessary.

Spring Roll Vegetable Wrap
Ingredients:
1 Jicama
1 Zucchini
1 Small head of cabbage
2 Heirloom Tomatoes
Raw sprouted hummus
1 Avocado, cut in chunks
Spring roll paper

Directions: Shred jicama, zucchini, and cabbage and mix together. Soak the spring roll paper until soft and pliable. Spread thin layer of hummus on spring roll paper. Add the shredded vegetable mix. Place tomatoes and avocado on top. Roll all ingredients in the paper. Enjoy.

Nori Vegetable Wrap
Ingredients:
1 Jicama
1 Zucchini
1 Red Bell Pepper
1 Handful sunflower seed sprouts
1 Cucumber
2 Heirloom Tomatoes
1 Jalepeño
1 Avocado, cut in chunks
Namu Shoyu or Organic Tamari or Coconut Aminos
Nori roll paper

Directions: Slice jicama, zucchini, bell pepper and cucumber thinly. Chop the tomatoes, jalepeño and avocado. Place the thinly sliced vegetables, tomato, jalepeño and avocado along one edge of the nori roll paper. On the opposite edge, place the Namu Shoyu, Tamari or Coconut Aminos. Roll the vegetables up in the nori wrap, sealing the opposite edge. Cut in bite sized pieces. Enjoy.

Coconut Yogurt
Ingredients:
2 cups young thai coconut
1 cup rejuvelac
½ cup lemon juice

Directions: Add all ingredients to blender and process until smooth. Enjoy as is, or add any variety of fresh fruit.

Chia Pudding
Ingredients:
1 1/2 cups nut milk or coconut milk
1/3 cup chia seeds
1/2 tsp. vanilla
2 Tbsp. maple syrup or honey (optional)

Directions: Add all ingredients in a jar, shake vigorously and place in refrigerator. Let chill for an hour and shake vigorously again. Chill for another 2 hours or more. Enjoy as is, or add any variety of fresh fruit, nuts, chai spice (see below) or cinnamon.

Chai Spice
Ingredients:
1 tsp Cardamon
Pinch Powdered Ginger
Pinch Cinnamon
Pinch Powdered Black Pepper
Pinch Powdered Star Anise
Pinch Powdered Clove

Directions: Mix all ingredients thoroughly.

Banana Ice Cream
5 Frozen Bananas - Peel and chop banana into bite sized pieces before freezing

Directions: Once bananas are frozen, place in K-Tek blender along with 1 tsp. chai spice. Add more or less chai spice to taste. Enjoy.

Chocolate Pudding
Ingredients:
1 ripe Avocado
1/4 cup Pitted Dates
1/4 cup Raw Cacao Powder
1/4 cup Nut Milk
1 tsp. Vanilla

Directions: Put everything in a food processor or K-Tek blender. Blend for 15 seconds, scrape down the side and blend again until thoroughly mixed and smooth. Chill for 30 minutes. Enjoy.

Exercise

I hope this Chapter has caused you to think about food a bit differently. For example, Week 1, you may want to practice gratitude for your meal. Week 2 you may want try a new recipe each week, etc.

Follow this link to download the 60-Day Anti-Aging Body Master Plan worksheet to help you track and create your personalized Master Plan. By writing out your thoughts and ideas, you will be designing your blueprint for success!

http://goo.gl/E5FFMj

CHAPTER ELEVEN

60 Days to a Sexier, Younger, Healthier New YOU!

"The secret of change is to focus all of your energy, not on fighting the old, but on building the new."

~Socrates

"If you do not change direction, you may end up where you are heading."

~Lao Tzu

Pulling It All Together

I hear all the time "Change is hard!" I believe that change is a decision and a mindset. Think about all the different things you have dedicated yourself to: parenting, education, a sport, a relationship, a job. Yes, anything you dedicate yourself to takes effort. But, the end result is rewarding. And, the process can be FUN!

It is the same with your health. It can be challenging, but the rewards are well worth the effort. Imagine a life where you don't need medication, where you have the energy to do the things you love, where you feel good, look sexier and younger! All this and more is within your reach.

I was one of the most unlikely people to change their diet. I liked white bread, fried potatoes, my mom's spaghetti - and dessert! I did not like where my health was headed. I decided to incorporate truly healthy foods, crowding out the bread and pasta. I tried new things and found I really enjoyed a salad. I discovered raw chocolate. It wasn't until later that I discovered that my tastebuds changed and I truly no longer liked tortillas and chips. It no longer took willpower to chose fresh fruit over a chocolate cake.

I made new associations with food. I felt alive and vibrant after eating a spinach salad with all the fixings. If I tried some mashed potatoes and gravy, I felt dead and lethargic. I know that if I was able to make those new associations, you can too!

If you have taken the time to work the exercises at the end of the chapters, incorporating new things over time, change becomes easy - especially when you see results!

There is a reason I ask clients to change one thing a week. It gives them time to master that change. I have found that if I try to change one thing, it is easy. If I try to change 15 things at once, I become overwhelmed and the change is not permanent. At the end of 8 weeks, 60 days, you will look and feel better!

ABOUT THE AUTHOR

Nikki Jeannine Stewart, Esq. CNHP, DHS, is an attorney, health educator, food advocate, certified yoga instructor and mother of two grown children. Along with running a busy personal injury and criminal defense law practice, she helps busy professionals look and feel younger by overcoming stress and all types of addictions through nutrition, meditation and exercise.

Her belief is that your body has the innate wisdom to heal and reverse the degenerative aging process, given the proper nutrients and support.

She is the author of the Anti-Aging Body: 60 Days to a Younger, Sexier, Healthier YOU! Nikki has practiced a healthy balanced lifestyle for over 25 years, using food, meditation and yoga as medicine to heal and restore vitality to the body, mind and spirit.

GLOSSARY

Adipose tissue: loose connective tissue designed to store energy in the form of fat; also cushions and insulates the body. Excess adipose tissue is linked to blood sugar and lipid problems, increasing risk of Type 2 Diabetes and coronary heart disease.

Antioxidant: molecule that inhibits the oxidation of other molecules; may prevent or delay some types of cell damage

Astaxathin: is an antioxidant supplement that helps fight the signs aging and joint and skeletal health. Protects the skin from sun damage

Ayurvedic: Literally translated "medicine of life." Entirely holistic system where its adherents work to create harmony between the body, mind, and spirit. It is this balance that prevents illness, treats acute conditions, and contributes to a long and healthy life.

Bentonite clay: internal and external cleanser; composed of aged volcanic ash, it has the ability to produce an electrical charge when hydrated. Upon contact with fluid, its electrical components change, giving it the ability to absorb toxins. Known for its ability to absorb and remove toxins, heavy metals, impurities, and chemicals.

Black box warning: type of alert that appears on the package inserts for certain prescription drugs; it is the strongest warning that the FDA requires, and signifies that medical studies indicate that the drug carries a significant risk of serious or even life threatening adverse effects

Co-factors: a non-protein chemical compound that is bound to a protein and is required for the protein's biological activity

Contact dermatitis: condition in which the skin becomes red, sore, or inflamed after direct contact with allergens or irritants

Crohn's Disease: an inflammatory bowel disease; it causes inflammation of the lining of your digestive tract, which can lead to abdominal pain, severe diarrhea and even malnutrition

Dioxin: Poisonous chemical sometimes used in farming and industry. Known to alter liver function. Linked to impairment of the immune system, the developing nervous system, the endocrine system and reproductive functions. Categorized as a "known human carcinogen"

Enzyme: large biological molecules responsible for the thousands of metabolic processes that sustain life

Estrogenic: any of several steroid hormones produced chiefly by the ovaries and responsible for the development and maintenance of female secondary sex characteristics

Ethylene di-bromide: a colorless toxic liquid compound that is used chiefly as a fuel additive in leaded gasolines; it has been found to be strongly carcinogenic; formerly used as an agricultural pesticide

Excitotoxins (MSG): Substances, usually amino acids, that stimulate overstimulate neuron receptors. Neuron receptors allow brain cells to communicate with each other. When exposed to excitotoxins, they fire impulses at such a rapid rate that they become exhausted. Several hours later, these depleted neurons die. Particularly susceptible are the hypothalamus and temporal lobes - the parts of the brain that control behavior, emotions, onset of puberty, sleep cycles and immunity. They have no nutritional value and are nothing other than chemicals added to foods to make them 'tastier'

Ghee: class of clarified butter that originated in India and is commonly used in South Asian cuisine and ritual

Gingivitis: very common form of gum disease that causes irritation, redness and swelling of your gums; due to its mildness, you may not be aware that you have the condition; can lead to much more serious gum disease and eventual tooth loss

Glutathione: very small molecule that is found in every cell; it's the body's most important antioxidant. Critical to support the liver in its detoxification process

Glycemic index: provides a measure of how quickly blood sugar levels rise after eating a particular type of food; it estimated how much each gram of available carbohydrate in a food raises a person's blood glucose level following consumption of the food, relative to consumption of pure glucose

Glycerin: a colorless, odorless, viscous liquid that is used in pharmaceutical formulations

Inflammation: the body's attempt at self-protection; the aim being to remove harmful stimuli, including damaged cells, irritants, or pathogens

Lymph: fluid that circulates throughout the lymphatic system; formed when the interstitial fluid is collected through lymph capillaries

Methyl bromide: Soil and structural fumigant, ozone-depleting chemical used as a pesticide. Damages the central nervous system and respiratory system.

Myelin sheath: found around the axon of a neuron; allows impulses to transmit quickly and efficiently along the nerve cells.

Oxidation: the combination of a substance with oxygen; a reaction in which the atoms in an element lose electrons and the valence of the element is correspondingly increased

Phagocytize: to engulf and destroy bacteria or other foreign materials

Photo contact dermatitis: arises from interaction between UV radiation and a product that contains drugs or chemicals that are photosensitizing agents

Psyllium husk: a shrub-like herb that is most commonly found in India; a bulking fiber that when ingested it expands and forms a mass in the colon by drawing water in it; the husks are able to scrub the intestines clean and transport waste through the intestinal tract

Seitan: aka wheat meat, wheat gluten, or simply gluten; food made from gluten, the main protein of wheat;

Shilajit: considered the root of Ayurvedic medicine; thick, sticky tar-like substance that strengthen the immune system, fortify cells, and muscles, and can be used as an anti-oxidant, an anti-stressor, and anti-allergen, and an anti-asthmatic

SSRI: Selective Serotonin Reuptake Inhibitor; typically used as an antidepressant

Transglutaminase: aka Meat Glue; Some meat glues are produced through the cultivation of bacteria, while others are made from the blood plasma of pigs and cows, specifically the coagulant that makes blood clot.

Triclosan: antibacterial agent and preservative used in personal care (soap, toothpaste and deodorant) and home cleaning products; Linked to heart disease and heart failure; Disrupts thyroid function and hormone regulation; Registered as a pesticide.

Vasodilation: widening of blood vessels.

NOTES

www.ingramcontent.com/pod-product-compliance
Lightning Source LLC
Chambersburg PA
CBHW071134280326
41935CB00010B/1220